HELP YOURSELF TO
HEALTH

HELP YOURSELF TO HEALTH

EXERCISES THAT REALLY WORK FOR MEN AND WOMEN

ESTHER FAIRFAX
Foreword by Katie Boyle

Photographed by Stuart Macleod

MACDONALD AND JANE'S · LONDON

First published in Great Britain in 1978 by
Macdonald and Jane's Publishers Limited, Paulton House, 8 Shepherdess Walk, London N.1

Copyright in the text © Esther Fairfax 1978
Copyright in the photographs © Macdonald and Jane's 1978
Design by David Fordham

CASED: ISBN 0 354 04283 1
LIMP: ISBN 0 354 04296 3

Filmset and printed in Great Britain by
BAS Printers Limited, Over Wallop, Hampshire

CONTENTS

FOREWORD	7
INTRODUCTION	9
HOW TO USE THIS BOOK	12
EXERCISES	
WARMING-UP	13
THE NECK AND CHIN	21
UPPER ARMS AND BOSOM	27
THE SHOULDERS	33
THE BACK	45
THE STOMACH	55
THE STOMACH AND THIGHS	67
THE THIGHS	83
THE BOTTOM	95
THE LEGS	107
ANKLES AND FEET	115
ARTHRITIS	121
POSTURE	125

To my husband John,
and my sons Michael and Jonathan.
They're magic.

FOREWORD

Letters flow in by the hundreds each week onto my *Dear Katie* desk at the TV Times, and I try to tackle most of the problems they contain constructively. But one subject had me foxed for ages – spot reducing: the people who asked 'How do I lose weight just where I want to?'

I put those into a 'pending' folder and hoped that one day I'd find the answer. I did. The day I met Esther Fairfax. I watched her in action, and I spoke to some of her pupils who were starry-eyed about the success of her methods.

Then I asked Esther whether she couldn't put some of these into black and white? 'I don't see why not,' she replied cautiously. I pushed a little: 'For instance, is there anything to be done to firm flabby upper arms?' 'Oh, yes, that's easy!' said Esther (see page 28).

After that I pulled out my pending file, picked a letter and printed it and Esther's suggestion – the response was enormous and Esther Fairfax solved this and many other similar problems which had piled up.

So you see, I like to think this book is in part a result of our meeting. Because I know how many people have already benefited tremendously from Esther's teaching methods, I'm quite sure a lot more can do so with this little book.

KATIE BOYLE

I wish to thank Kit Barker for giving me the title of this book, and also his wife, Ilse, for her optimism and enthusiastic encouragement. **E.F.**

INTRODUCTION

HELP YOURSELF TO HEALTH

We all want to be really fit and full of energy, and yet most of us neglect that vital ingredient to perfect health—exercise! That word may conjure up visions of hours of physical jerks or energetic sport, but it need not be so drastic. Exercising can be fun, as well as beneficial, as I hope you'll agree when you've tried the exercises in this book.

Exercise is a natural requirement of the human body. The stretch and yawn most of us indulge in first thing in the morning is the body demanding exercise after a night's comparative inactivity—although, if you've ever seen one of those speeded-up films of someone sleeping, you'll have noticed just how much the sleeper tosses and turns. The body needs almost continual movement, and even when we are deeply asleep and relaxed we move, because we *need* to move.

And these needs are very easy to uncover. Think of what happens on a long car journey: after driving for four hours non-stop, you feel exhausted and drained of energy; if you stopped and got out, had a little walk, flexed your muscles and had a little skip and jump (if you didn't feel too silly doing it!), you would recharge your energy banks, regain concentration and ease your tension—and no doubt that of your passengers! Similarly, you will have felt the loss of energy and concentration that comes with sitting at a desk or in front of the television continuously for an hour or so. You should really get up every 15 to 20 minutes and have a stretch and walk around which recharges you and keeps your joints and muscles from locking too long in one position.

Most people who participate occasionally in medium to strenuous exercise are surprised by their feeling of well-being afterwards. Instead of the anticipated exhaustion, they feel less tired and are invigorated instead. It is an indisputable fact that each and every body needs a certain amount of exercise to keep it going and healthy. Doing too little rather than too much saps energy, but equally, doing *too* much isn't much help (don't, for instance, rush about cleaning the house before guests arrive: you'll only be tired and bad-tempered instead of enjoying them as you should). Rest should be as much part of your fitness programme as exercise: combined, they calm your nerves, refresh you, and give you more vitality.

Low mental states, too, like unhappiness or depression, can alter your metabolism, so that you feel a real, positive tiredness. There are actual chemical changes in your brain, but this can be remedied by about ten minutes exercise, which releases a chemical in the body closely related to antidepressants. So, no matter how awful you feel—tired, bored, lethargic, depressed, completely cast-down—you should force yourself to do something really energetic: dance wildly to some pop music, run round the garden until you're breathless, run upstairs instead of walking, walk everywhere briskly, not quite breaking into a run. Minutes later, you'll feel entirely different, full of bounce and energy, ready to face or tackle everything and anything.

THE HEART OF THE MATTER

Your heart is the most important muscle in your body. It is a muscular bag roughly the size of a closed fist, which runs continuously and without servicing for a lifetime, all the while pushing out eighty gallons of blood an hour. If for any reason the heart cannot pump as much blood as the tissues require, cells all over the body will suffer oxygen starvation and will be less able to function efficiently.

The best 'service' you can give to your heart is exercise, because no matter what exercise you take, the effects on the body are the same—your joints move, your muscles contract and lengthen, your lungs operate at full capacity, your pulse rate is raised through exercise, the heart becomes a better and more efficient energy conserver. This means that the oxygen or energy demands on the heart are lower, and the result is that the heart functions efficiently. It can cope with the demands made on it during your daily life and the stress therein.

Exercising your heart can extend your life. Those who undertake regular and vigorous exercise considerably reduce their chances of developing heart problems: in fact heart attacks are twice as common among office workers as they are among manual workers. And there is plenty of evidence to show that people with hypertension can lower their blood pressure through wise use of exercise.

An under-exercised heart is likely to make you feel lethargic and lacking in energy. It will require firm and constant exercise to revitalize it. So you should begin any exercise regime gently and work your heart and pulse rate up by regular exercise for a few minutes each day.

But most importantly, before throwing yourself into any form of exercise, please be sensible and talk to your doctor first, to check that you are not going to endanger yourself in any way. If you have a particularly severe weight problem, for instance, suffer from high blood pressure, or are being treated by drugs, you should seek medical advice as to whether such physical activities are recommended.

KEEP YOUR PANTS UP!

And this is what is so vital to the whole principle of your health and your heart. The acceleration of the pulse rate which is the result of exercise promotes efficiency of the heart, the lungs, and all the muscles and manifests itself in vigorous breathing—*pants*.

A fifteen-minute unbroken exercise programme should be undertaken each day. That's the optimum. Otherwise at least enough exercise should be taken so that you become breathless and raise the pulse rate. You should, indeed *must*, work up a pant!

Begin gently if you've never done any form of exercise before, or haven't exercised for a long time. You can increase your effort thereafter bit by bit as you build up stamina and breathlessness until you can cope with a really good pant. There is a great difference between gasping for breath and panting, and you shouldn't work yourself to the point of gasping, nor to a stage when you feel your heart pound in your head instead of in your chest. Should this occur, you're over-extending yourself and probably extremely out of condition. You are certainly not yet ready to cope with vigorous fitness exercises. Start even more gently with a daily brisk walk, then a gentle run of about 25 to 30 metres. This will get your pants up.

If you decide that jogging is for you, jog for a while then walk for a bit, jog, walk, and so on. And that way of working could well and sensibly apply to the way we live our lives. If it is all hustle and bustle we'll surely end the day exhausted and tense. It shouldn't be beyond us, and certainly would benefit us, to strike a balance between rest and work in all our activities.

It is of no real advantage if you do not

exercise regularly. When you have a sedentary job, a sudden burst of enthusiastic exercising, and then nothing else, is like going on a crash diet. You will see little result, do yourself no good, and most likely will feel ghastly and give it up as a lost cause. Just do a little each day, get your pants up, and you will find that exercise is like a generator—the more you put into it, the more energy you have.

The joy of life, the richness it holds, are heightened by our health and well-being. It is all free. All you need is a little disciplined exercise each and every day.

Keep your pants up!

THE SHAPE OF THINGS TO COME

We now know the right sort of exercise to keep our heart, lungs, and circulation in tip-top condition. The exercises presented in this book will benefit your health and vitality. Equally important, they are carefully designed to give your figure shape by firming-up flabby muscles and so will help you to look and feel youthful.

Let us first understand why we should, and must, exercise our muscles. We'll start simply with an exercise for your imagination. Stand tall and imagine that you are looking at yourself in a mirror. Strip off your clothes. If you are overweight, strip off the fat. And, under the skin, what a fantastic network of muscles you have. Now the crunch. If you strip every muscle, the bones will drop into a heap on the floor. All two hundred of them!

That's how important your muscles are. Your skeleton needs your muscles for every move you make, and to make all these movements efficiently, your muscles need to be in good condition. And this comes from the right sort of exercise, and from eating the right kind of food. It doesn't take a great deal of imagination to see that a sensible combination of exercise and healthy food will improve your figure and give you bags of vitality.

If you don't exercise, eat trashy foods, are overweight, you can expect to suffer from headaches, backache, nervous tension, lack of energy, tiredness. And if you already do, then it is high time you started to work on yourself. In fact, recent research has suggested that a concentrated half hour of exercise each day can help you lose at least half a pound in one week. This may not sound exciting, but in a year, you could lose a stone and a half without cutting out your favourite tipple or occasional treat—as well as doing every part of your body a lot of good!

First, diet. Do try to eat properly, preferably wholefoods. Your weight can so easily creep up the scales without your really noticing it, and it takes lots of effort and time to take weight off. Please keep away, too, from faddy diets. Before I learned about nutrition and exercise, I can remember weeks of misery when I failed yet again to lose weight after trying diet after diet. If you start to eat properly, your weight should reduce naturally, but do remember that you didn't become overweight, flabby or unfit overnight, so you can't expect results overnight. Above all don't let yourself become disheartened. In my twenties, for instance, I was extremely overweight, and used to weigh eleven stone. Now I delight in a trim seven and a half stone.

But the shape of things to come is also controlled by exercise. You should make looking after your body and your health a life-long activity, rather like keeping up insurance payments to reap rewards with a more lithe and lively middle and old age. As we become older our muscles tend to lose their elasticity, joints stiffen and agility can become something we used to have. There is really no reason for us to sit back and accept this. It is well worth investing time, patience and discipline *now*, so that you can achieve real fitness, and retain it. Make exercise a daily routine; if you can find time to eat at least one meal a day, you can spare at least 15 minutes for an exercise session which will do as much good.

It is not difficult, therefore, to see why our skeletons need us to stretch and strengthen our muscles; they're what keep us upright and take the strain off our joints, and we need to look after them.

HOW TO USE THIS BOOK

You will notice that the majority of exercises throughout this book are starred. This star system is an indication of the difficulty of the exercise, ranging from the relatively easy one star to tough exercises with five stars. A number of exercises have no stars, and these are ones which should be a basic ingredient of each and every exercise session you undertake. Using the no star exercises and low star rating will, however, build up your strength and stamina and enable you to tackle the higher star movements later on.

But the star system is also an aid to a varied exercise routine. You can work out your own exercise routines by choosing different stars each week, and by doing this you can keep boredom at bay, and use a greater variety of muscles at the same time. Choose exercises for each session as you would choose food from a menu, and make it more fun by doing the exercises to music.

You may feel stiff a day or two after first exercising if you're not used to it. This is quite natural and the best treatment is to keep to a regular graduated programme. As your muscles become accustomed to working you'll feel less stiffness and eventually none at all. By this time you will have built up stamina and should also notice your muscles firming up and your figure becoming shapely.

The Victorians thought they were old at forty. We say 'life begins at forty'. And I will happily vouch for that. I'm more fit, have more energy, feel more full of fun and life than I did in my twenties. I hope that by using my exercises, you too will be able to share in the fitness and well-being that we can all achieve. Don't let the natural vivacious vitality of youth become a mere memory.

Esther Fairfax
Hermitage, Berkshire
January 1978

WARMING UP

Before starting any exercise session it is sensible to begin with a few gentle warming-up exercises. They will make your joints more mobile and loosen up your muscles—essential if you're unfit or haven't been taking some sort of regular exercise; in fact they're essential as a safety measure, because an unused muscle can be pulled or even torn. They will also increase your circulation which will help feed your muscles with oxygen and blood, making them more willing to respond to the work they may not otherwise be ready to do. They will also raise your pulse rate, make your heart beat a bit faster, and start you panting!

WARMING UP I

Repeat this warming-up exercise several times until you feel that your body and joints are loosened up enough to start whatever exercise routine you have chosen to follow. Do it once a day at least.

1. Stand tall and straight with your arms stretched up to the ceiling. Keep your legs together.

Bend your knees. Let your head swing downwards, followed by your body and arms, curling your spine.

Bend your knees again as your arms and body swing up to full height. Finish as you began with your arms stretched up to the ceiling.

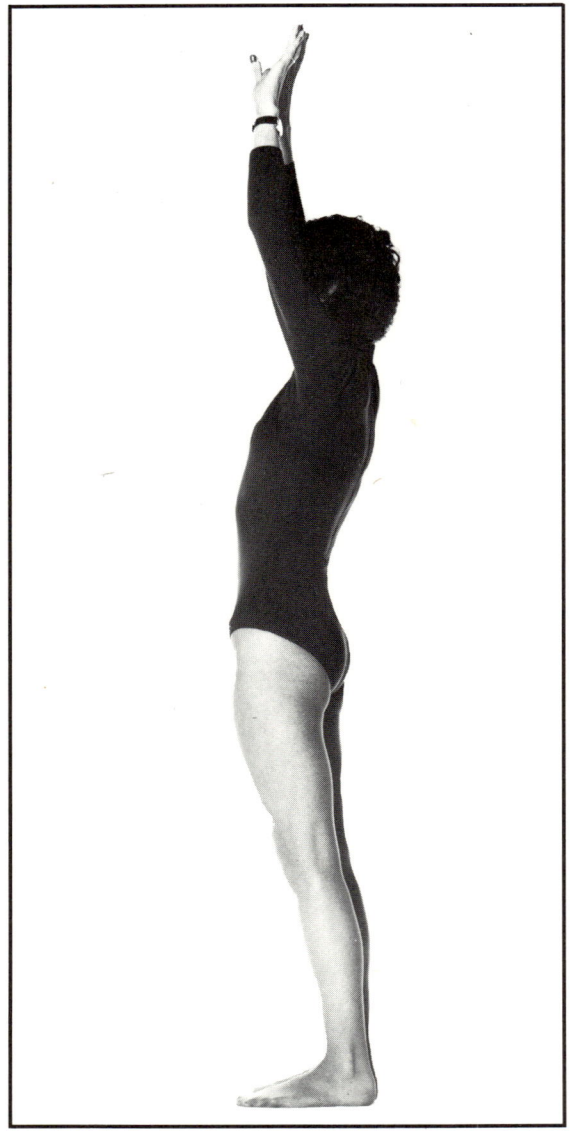

WARMING UP 15

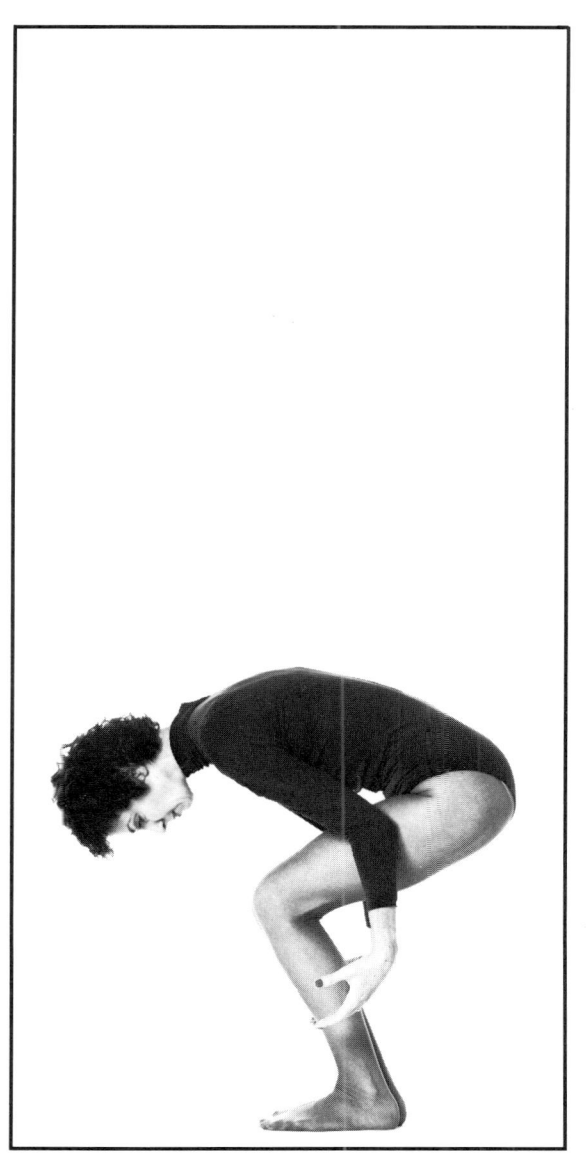
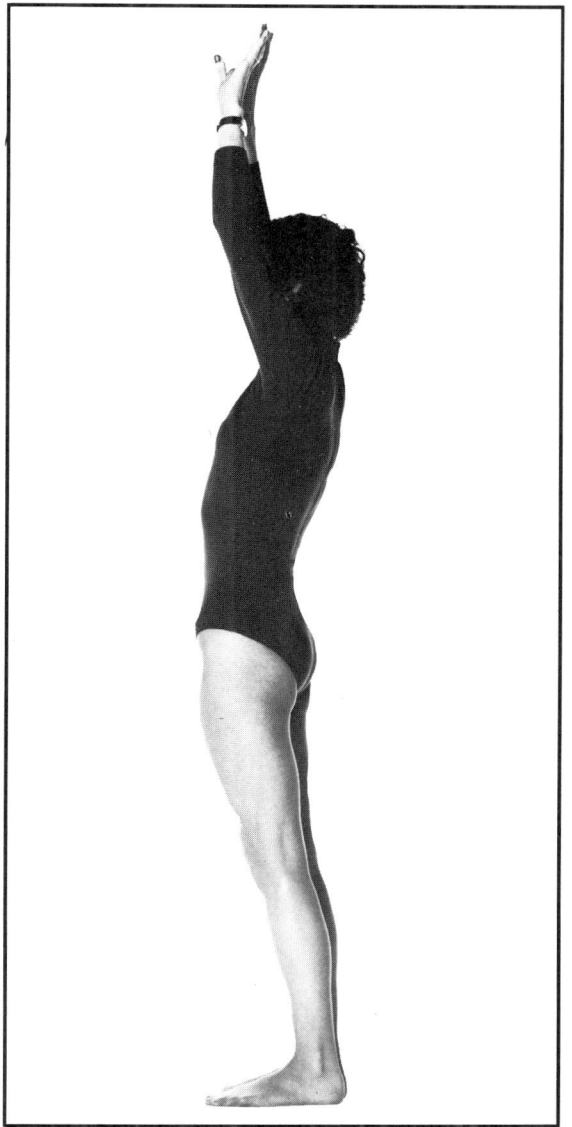

WARMING UP II

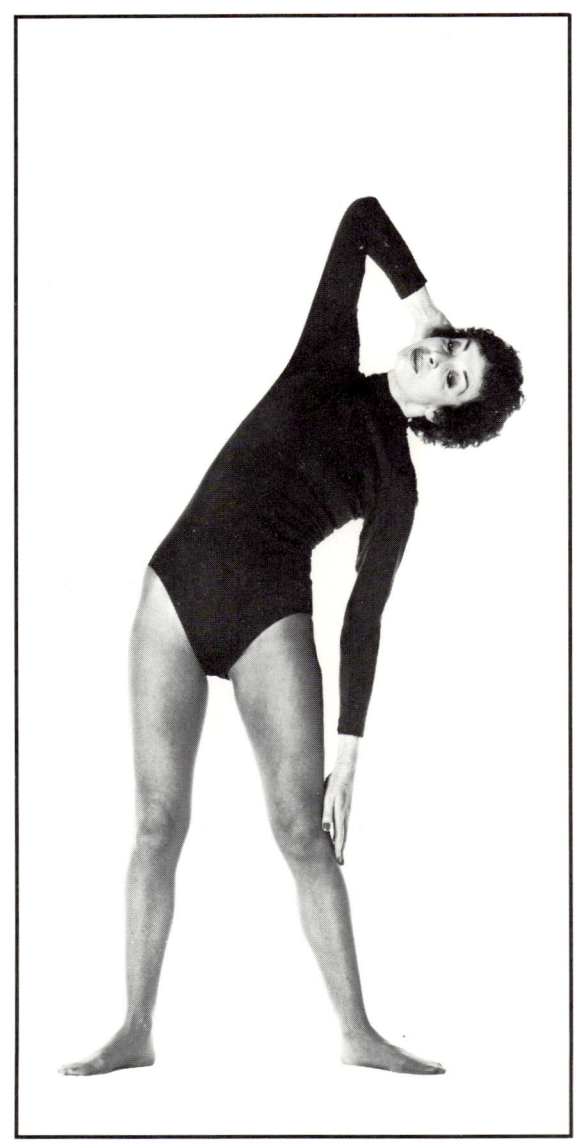

These warming-up exercises are particularly good for the waist. They really make your midriff muscles work by stretching them, thus hastening the firming-up process. But they can make you a little dizzy, so only do a few movements on each side to begin with. Gradually do a few more each day, until you can manage ten times on each side. Before long, you should notice your waistline becoming more shapely. But once a day is enough.

1. Stand with your feet apart. Place one hand behind your head and let your other arm hang loosely at your side so that it can slide down your outside leg. Don't allow your hip to lean or be pushed to one side. From your waist down, your body and legs should stay quite straight. Once in this position, pump over to one side several times.

Stand tall again. Change hands around, and pump over to the other side several times.

2. Stand tall. Place both your hands behind your head and gently swing over from side to side. Once again do please be sure your hips don't move so that the pull comes from your waist.

WARMING UP 17

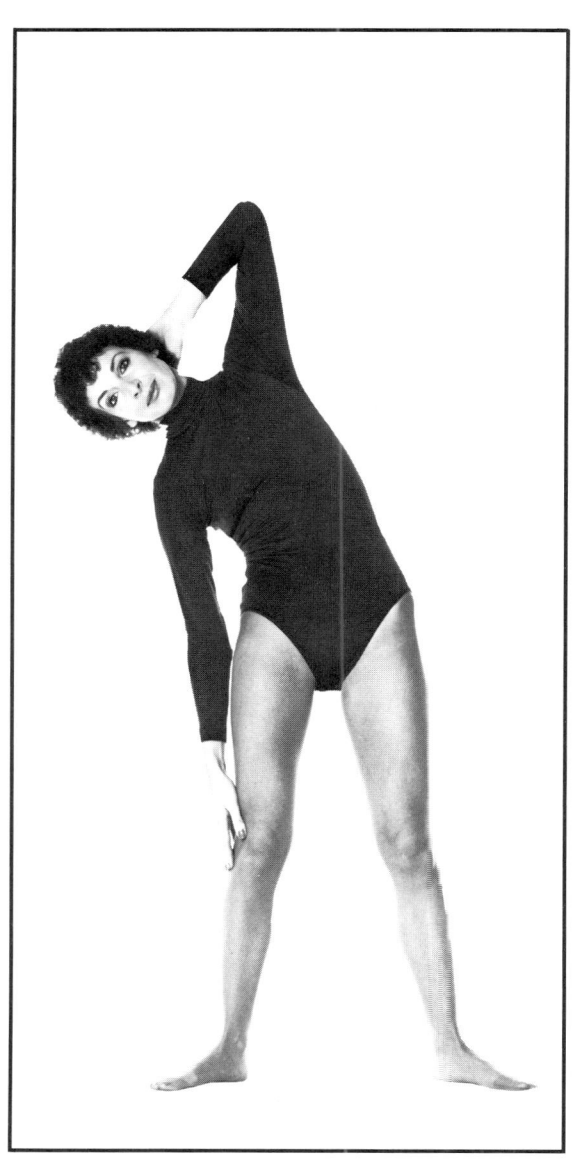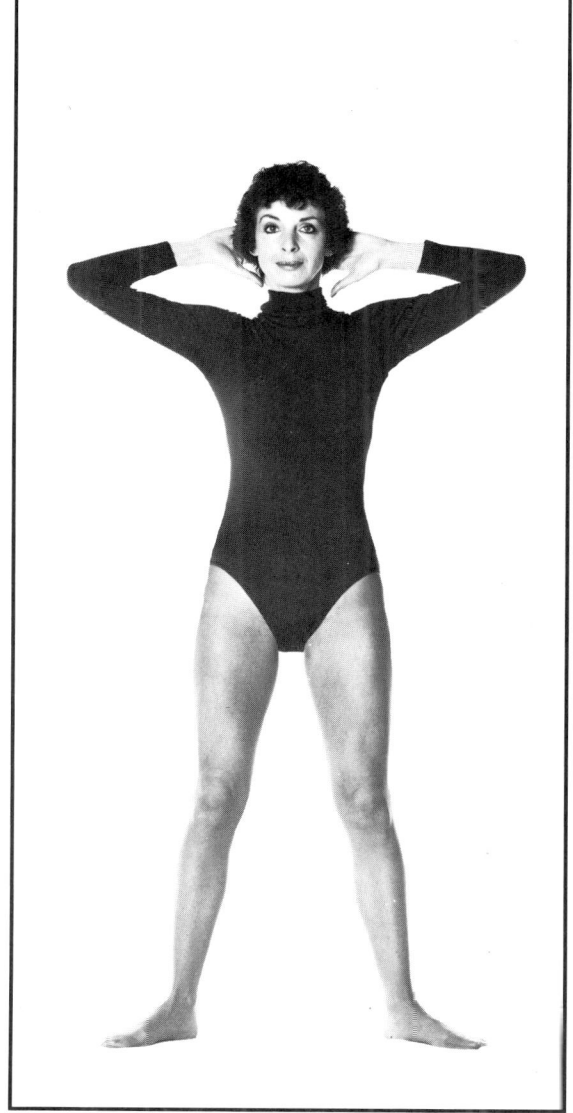

WARMING UP III

This warming-up exercise will get your circulation going and bring colour to your cheeks. But its main objective is to give you a lovely stretch through your spine and right down the backs of your legs. When these particular muscles lose their elasticity, that nice young bouncy walk can slow down and in years to come might turn into a shuffle-along crawl. So try to do this exercise at least once a day.

1. Stand with your legs apart and your arms stretched above your head.

Start lowering your body forward by sticking out your bottom and making a hollow along your spine like a racehorse. Hold this position for a slow count of five.

Next, *round* your back and allow your arms and your head to drop down towards the floor. Keep your legs straight.

Pump down as though you want to touch the floor with your hands—to the count of five—and you will feel the muscles in the back of your thighs working. Don't worry if you can't touch the floor at first—you'll be able to after practise.

Lastly while you are still down, pump your hands and arms through your legs as though you wanted to grab an imaginary tail. Push through five times.

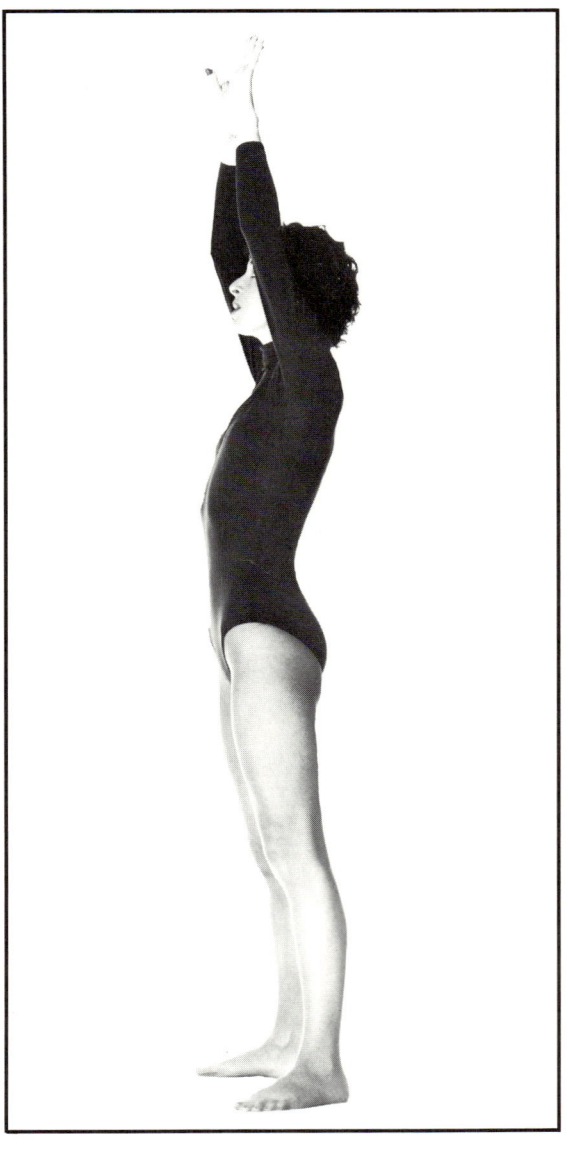

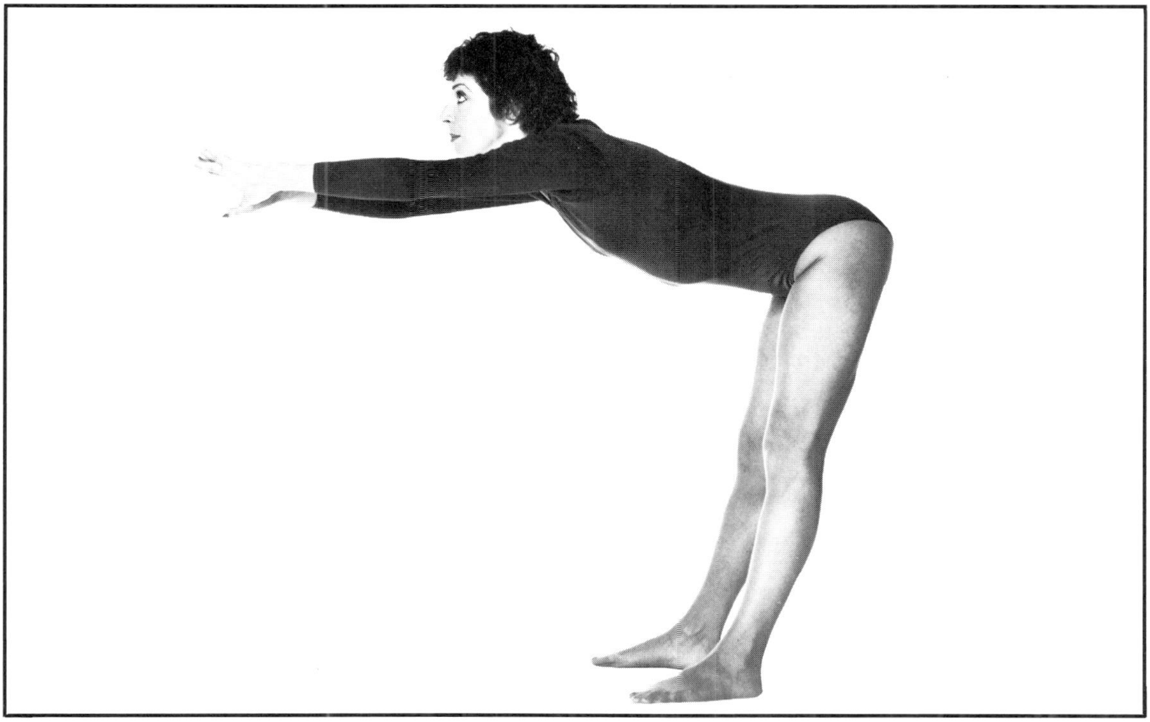

WARMING UP 19

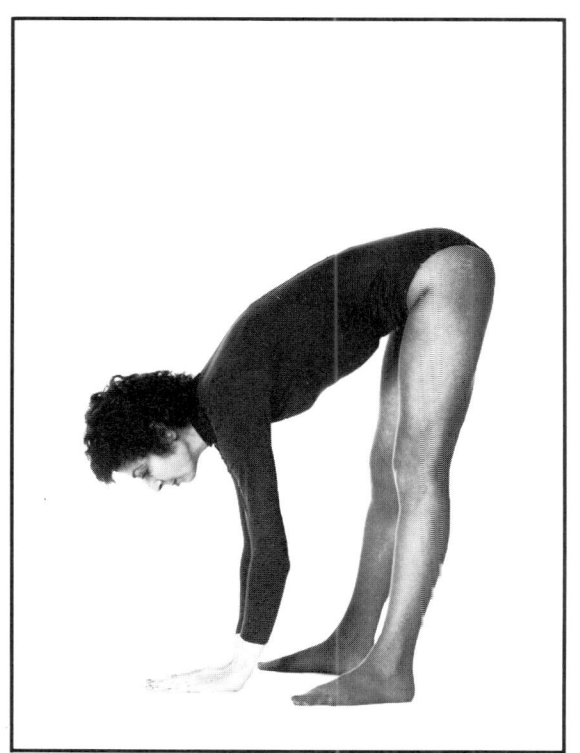
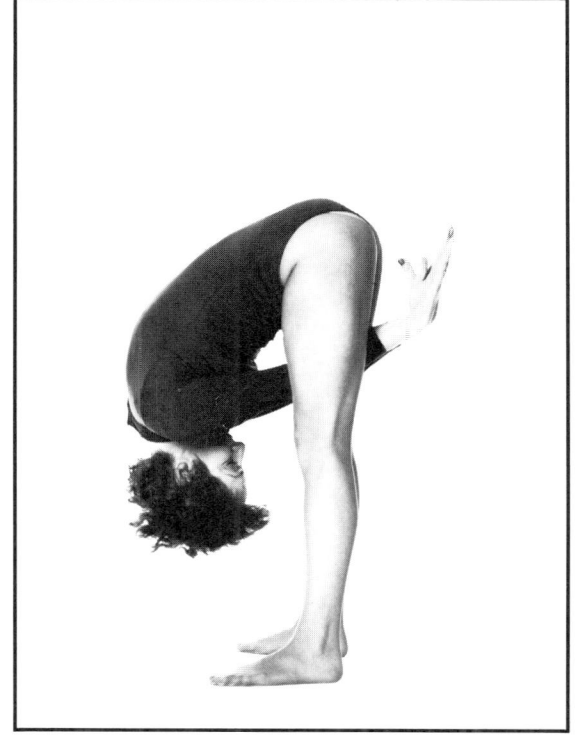

THE NECK AND CHIN

The neck and chin have also got muscles which can become slack and therefore unsightly. It is surprising how much a neck can be neglected, even though a daily facial beauty routine is followed; the neck is after all a continuation of your face and can benefit from exactly the same treatment—cleansing, massaging and moisturizing. It is often the neglected neck, allowed to become scraggy, that can betray age in an otherwise youthful body. Regular exercise to utilize the muscles can help alleviate any slackness.

THE NECK AND CHIN I

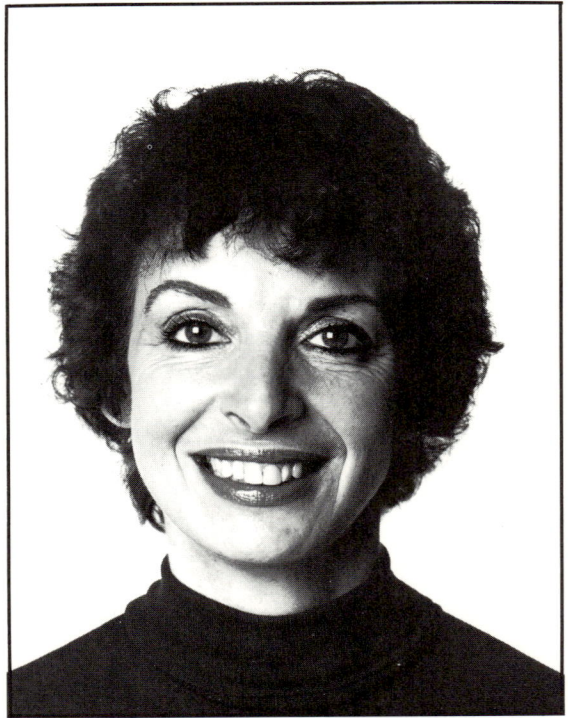

Do these exercises in front of a mirror at first—preferably on your own as you won't be a pretty sight! When you've practised them a few times, you will be able to do them anywhere at anytime. I often do them while sitting in the car in traffic jams or at lights, and get some very startled looks!

1. Begin smiling. Grin hard. While you are grinning widely with all teeth showing turn down the corners of your mouth as hard as you can so that your grin becomes a hideous grimace. You should now look as though you're taking the lead in a horror film, with all the muscles in your neck standing out visibly. Hold this grimace for a count of five. Relax. Then do it all again.

Repeat this exercise as often as you like, but certainly try to do it at least once a day. It helps to stretch and firm the neck muscles and helps stop that slack appearance of the skin.

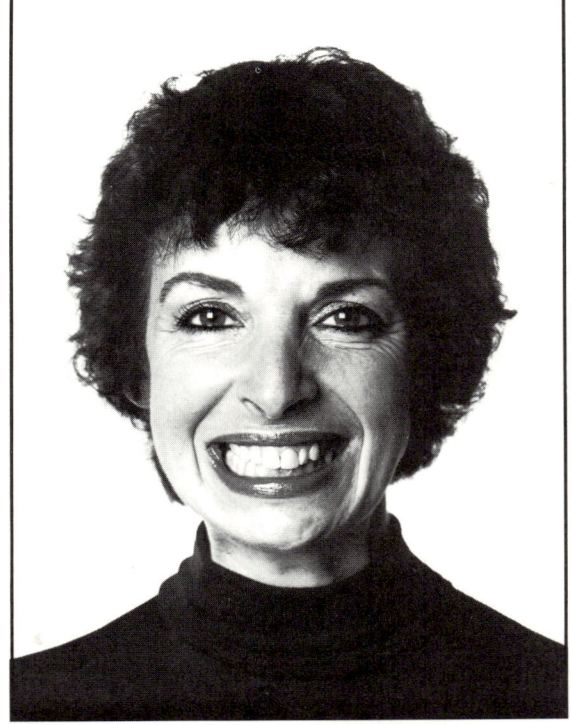

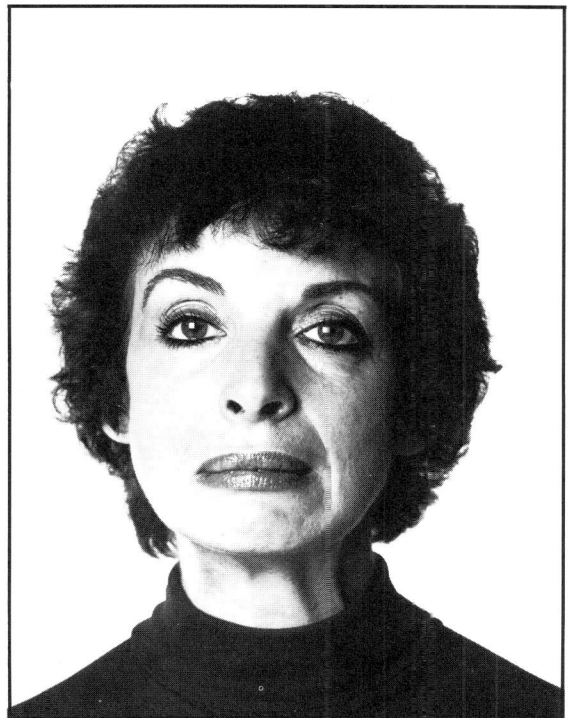
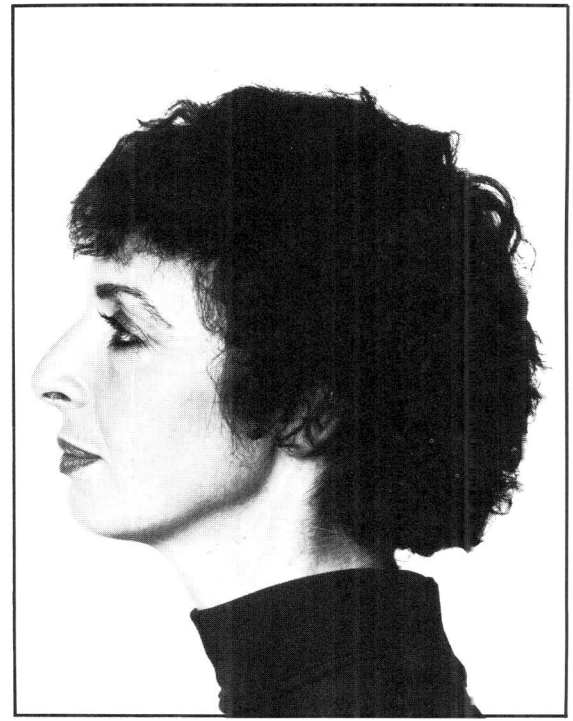

2. This exercise is one for the chin as well. Push your jaw forward and upward, lifting your lower lip up and over your upper lip as though it were straining to reach your nose. (I hope you don't succeed in reaching that high with your lower lip as it just wouldn't be normal!) Put a lot of effort into it, and it will stretch and firm all those muscles.

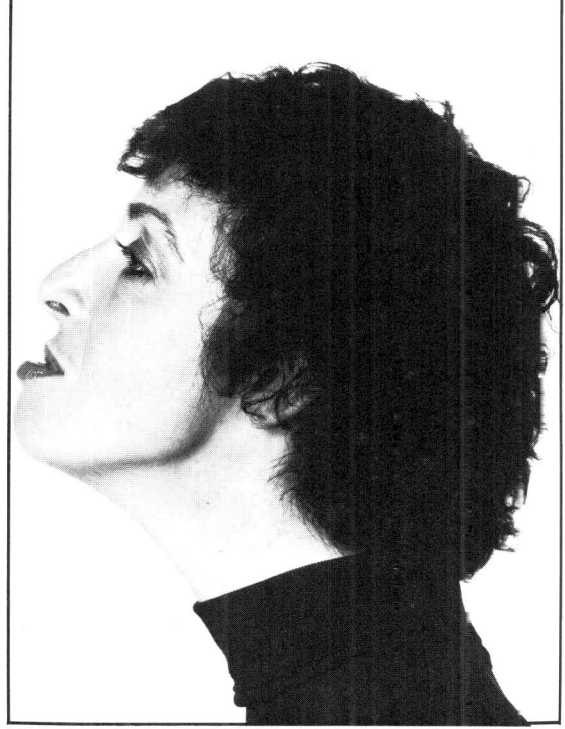

THE NECK AND CHIN II

Do this exercise frequently, and it will help tone up the muscles of the throat, and keep the chin and jaw firm. It is also relaxing, relieving tension at the back of the neck, vital for those of you with sedentary occupations.

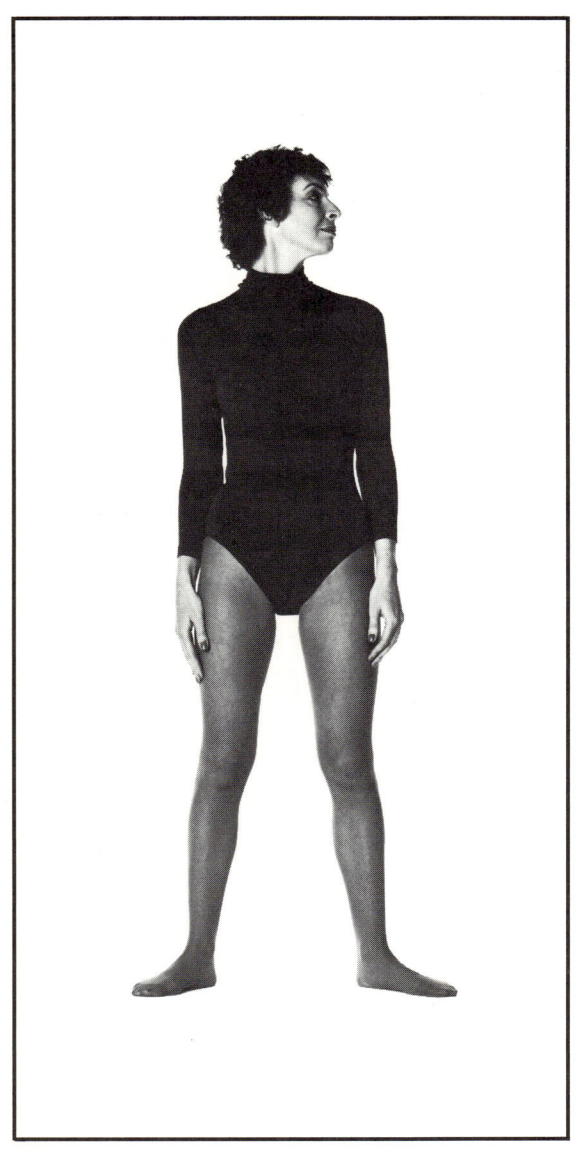
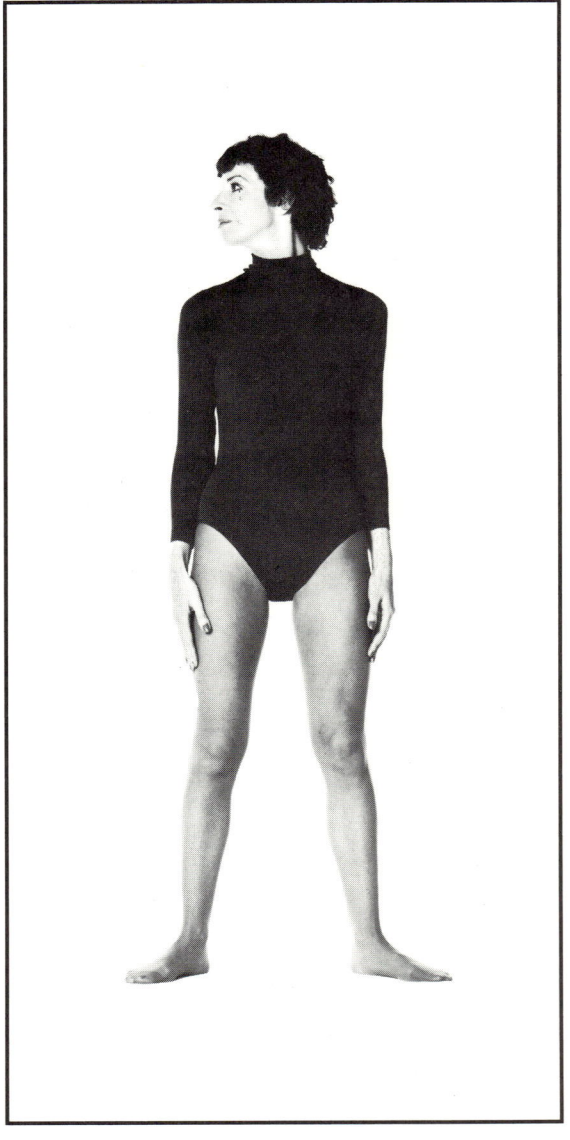

THE NECK AND CHIN

1. Turn your head slowly to your left until your chin is in line with your shoulder.

Gently turn your head round to look over your right shoulder. Try to look as far behind you as possible, but don't force it.

Look straight ahead. Raise your chin up, keeping your mouth closed, and stretch your head back as far as you can, to give yourself a really good stretch through and up your neck.

Lower your head until your chin rests on your chest. Do this whole exercise gently but firmly.

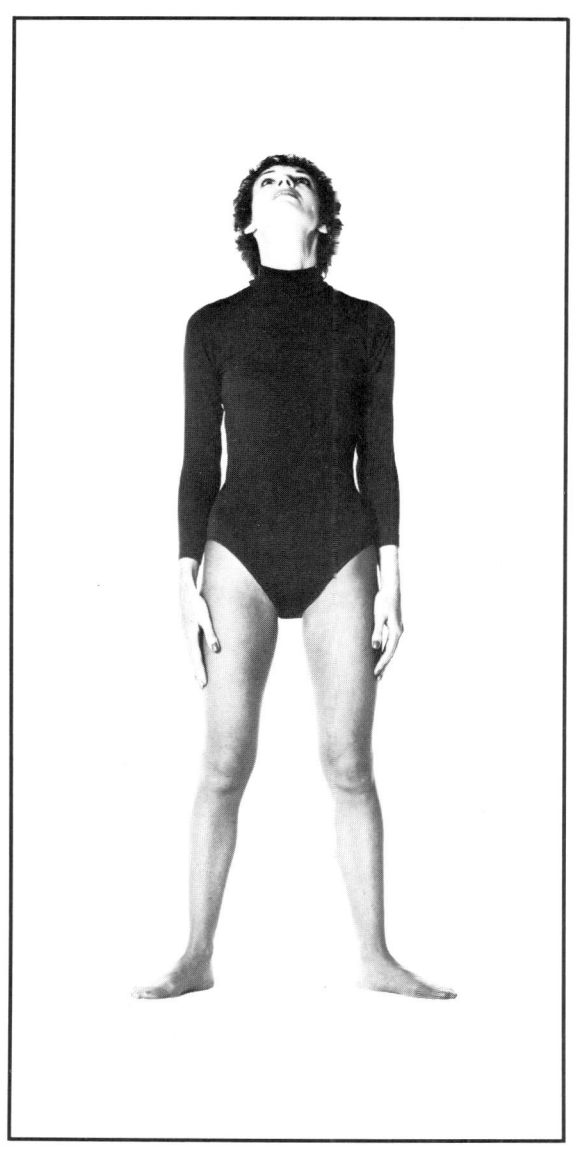

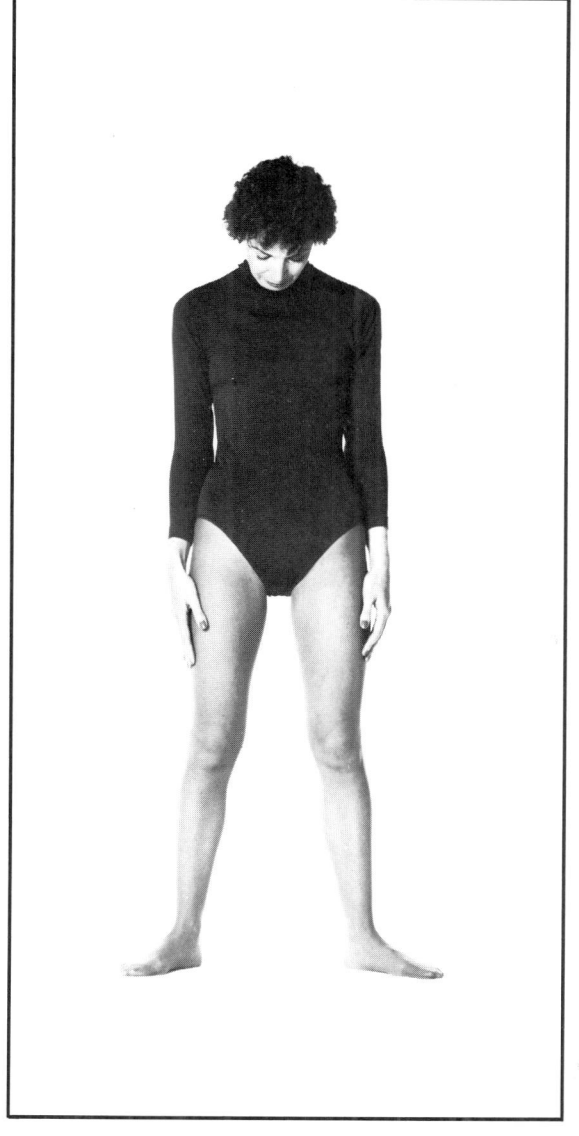

UPPER ARMS AND BOSOM

Flabby upper arms and drooping bosoms are two of the most vulnerable and troublesome areas for the majority of women. Both are caused by weak muscle tone, due to the fact that most of us don't use these muscles in everyday jobs or activities. The bosom, of course, consists of fibrous tissue and fat, with no actual muscle, but there is a muscle at the front of the arm pit—the pectoral muscle—which if exercised hard and frequently can at least prevent some slack and droop.

UPPER ARMS AND BOSOM I

Flabby upper arms can be particularly unsightly if you are overweight, and I know some women feel embarrassed by this, especially when they wear sleeveless dresses. It hardly needs mentioning that if you *are* overweight you could really help the problem by following a sensible wholefood diet which, coupled with this exercise, can help shape and firm up the neglected muscles.

1. Stand up straight, feet slightly apart, giving yourself plenty of room. Either clench your fists or hold an apple or orange firmly in your hands. Lift your arms to shoulder height and stretch out from either side of your body. It is important that while you do this exercise you keep your arms perfectly straight. Don't allow them to bend at all.

Start off making small circles with your arms. Check that you are not allowing your wrist to twist or turn and that your arms from shoulder to fist are still ramrod straight otherwise you will lose the value of the exercise.

Once you've got the idea, speed up your small circles. Keep your arms in a nice taut line and get those circles going faster. Count a slow five while your arms are going at top speed and then relax. Repeat this exercise as often as you like during the day. It's so easy to do and can be done almost anywhere.

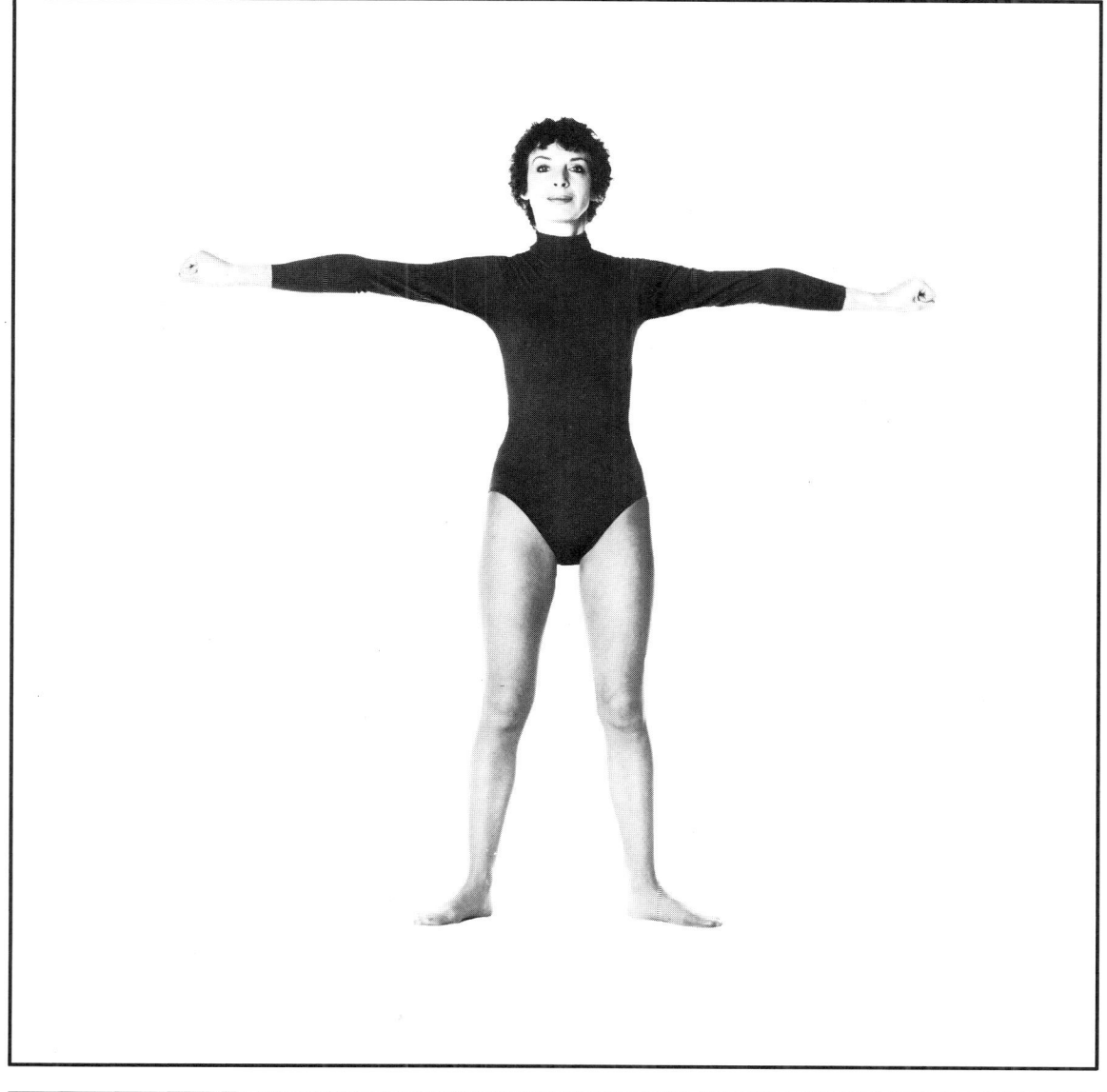

UPPER ARMS AND BOSOM II

Most women I talk to are unhappy about their bosoms—they're too large, too small, or they droop. Besides plastic surgery there is very little we can do unless we exercise the pectoral muscle which should give the bosom a little lift and make it appear firmer. Because the bosom is made up of fatty tissue, weight plays a part in its size. There are some women lucky enough to be born with just the right size and shape for their figures; meanwhile for all the rest of us it is a good idea to do this exercise as often as possible!

1. Grip your forearms with your hands as illustrated. Lift your arms and keep them at shoulder height. Grip very firmly and *push*, as if you were pushing your sleeves up. Your hands mustn't move, but you will push the skin up your arms.

If you do this exercise in front of a mirror you should be able to see the pectoral muscle jump up and stand out, and your bosom lift with every push. Start with ten pushes a day.

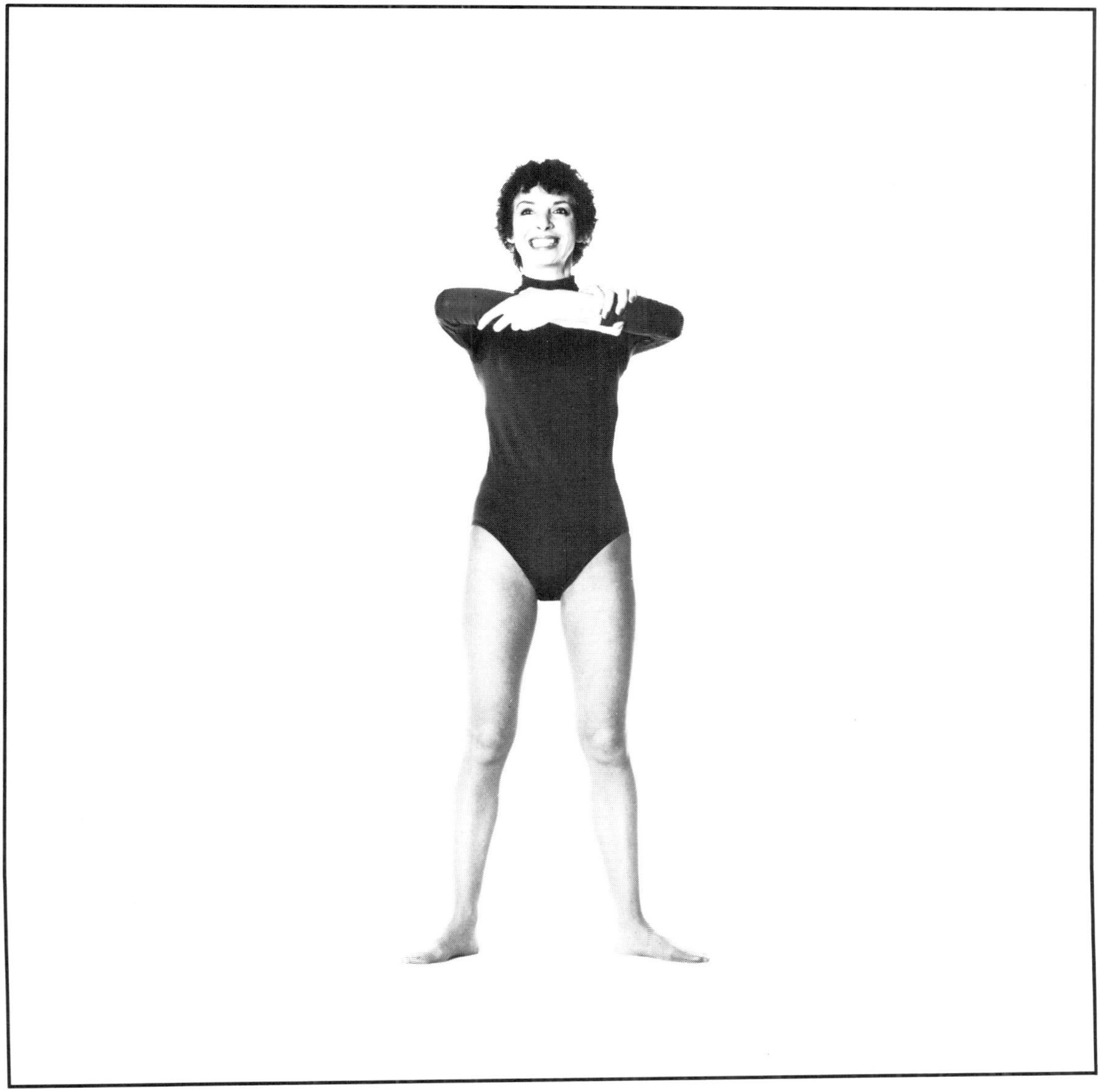

UPPER ARMS AND BOSOM 31

THE SHOULDERS

The shoulders are a problem area for everyone—men, women and children—principally because of bad posture. The sedentary nature of the majority of jobs can help develop a variety of problems, most notably what is called the 'dowager's hump'. This hump consists of fibro-fatty tissue that has gathered at the base of the neck between the central and upper part of the shoulder blades. Sometimes this tissue also forms at the buttocks, hips or thighs, occasionally even causing pain. A hump is most likely to develop, however, if you are overweight, mostly affects women who are middle aged or post-menopausal (it *can* affect men as well, though), but can be improved and eliminated by a combination of better posture, sensible diet, and plenty of vigorous daily exercise. I know of one woman of middle age who lost her hump after two years' perseverance with her exercises. That may seem rather a long time, but the time and effort involved were as nothing compared to her regained looks and confidence.

The shoulders are also an area connected with tension, which tends to gather at the base of the neck and across the shoulders, and these exercises can help alleviate a day's tension marvellously, if done in the evening or before going to bed. They also work wonders after a long car journey, which is one of the simplest and commonest causes of tension.

THE SHOULDERS I

The exercises on the next few pages are good for both dowager's hump, and for alleviating tension.

A dowager's hump can develop because of bad posture, so if you sit or walk round-shouldered, with your head in a forward and outward position, *don't*, and if you sleep with two pillows I suggest you try to sleep with one.

1.* Lift your shoulders as though you want them to touch your ears. Hold the position. Relax. Then lift your shoulders up again. Relax. Leave your hands and arms resting in your lap if you are sitting, or down by your sides if standing. Repeat this exercise until you feel you are becoming more relaxed and the tension is less. You can do it watching television, sitting in a car, almost anywhere.

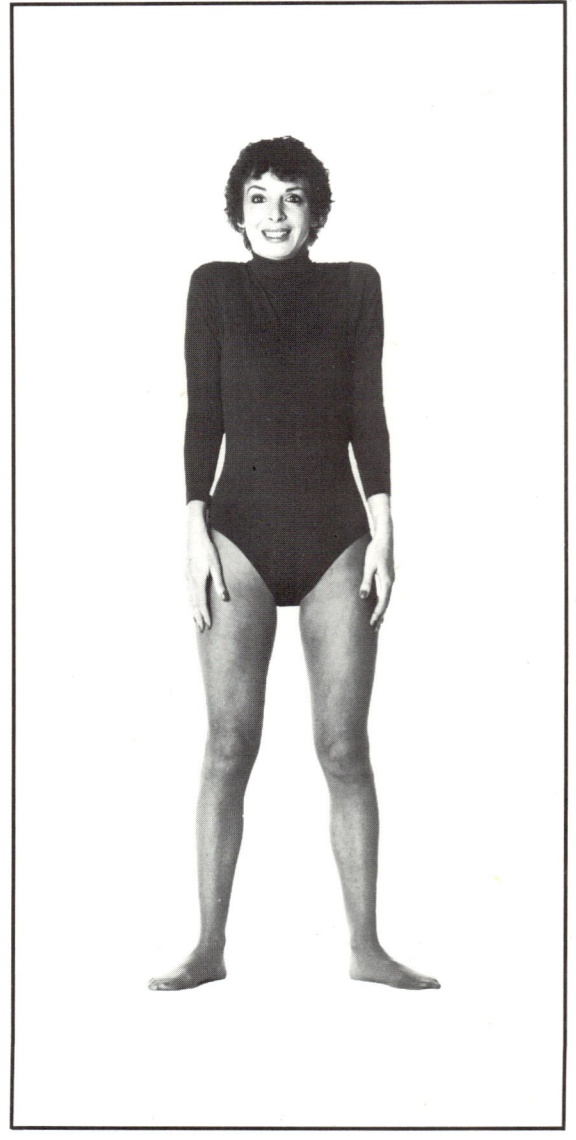

THE SHOULDERS 35

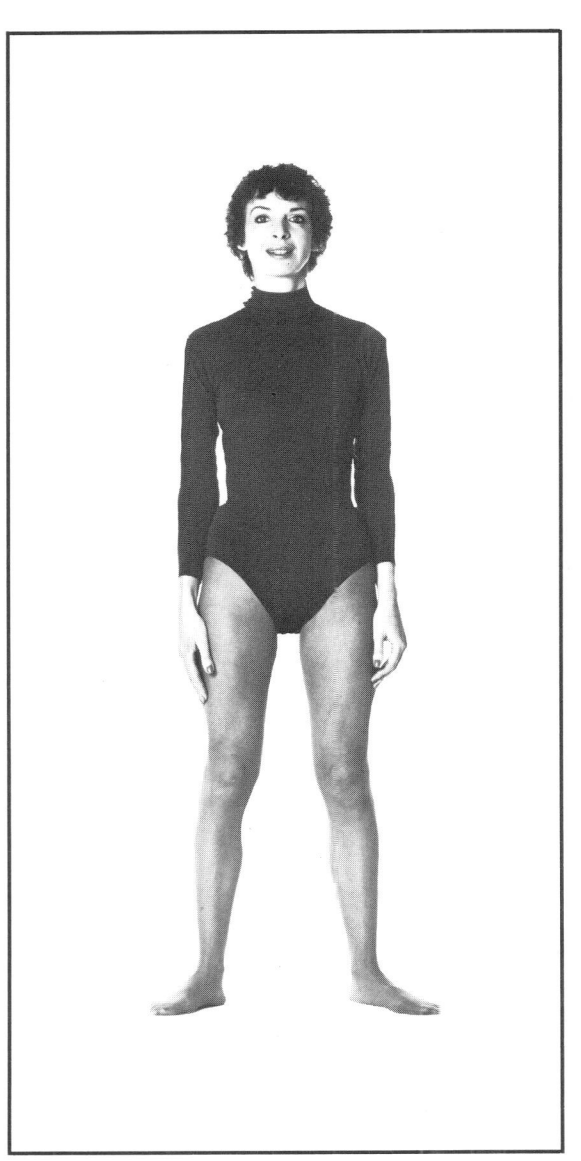 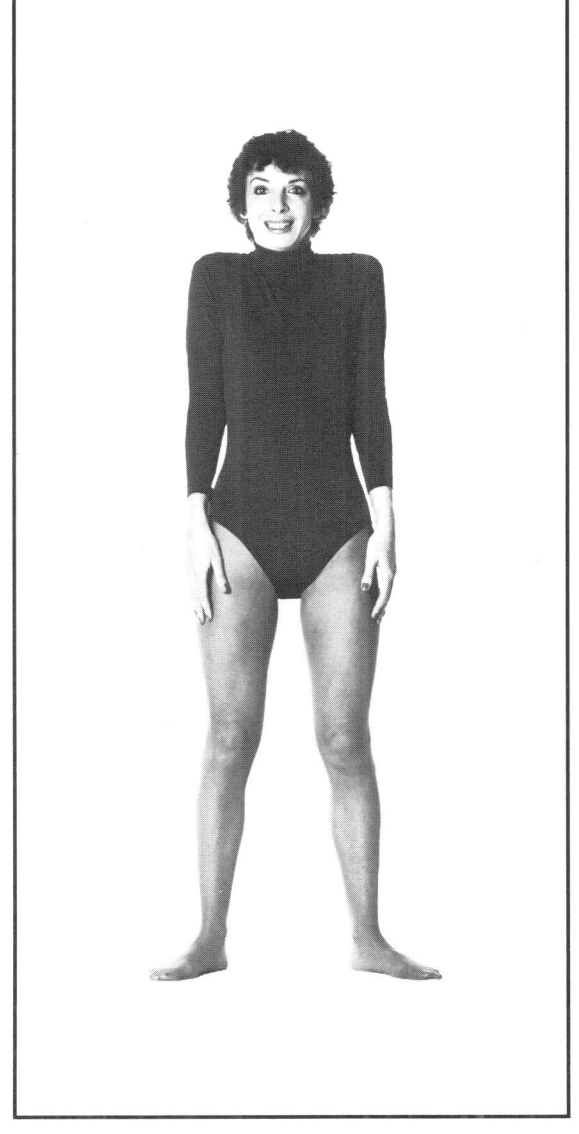

THE SHOULDERS II

1.* Place your hands on your shoulders and make large circles with your elbows. Keep your hands on your shoulders all the time. Bring your elbows forward and together. Try to make them touch in front of you if you can. Then bring them up and round in a big circle and as you bring them back be sure you really push back hard so that your shoulder blades are pushed together. Now down again and in front. Keep making a big circle while pushing back and round as you go. Repeat circles five times.

The pushing back and making your shoulders move against the hump or the tension, should help to prevent, even in time break down, the fatty tissues that can collect across the shoulders.

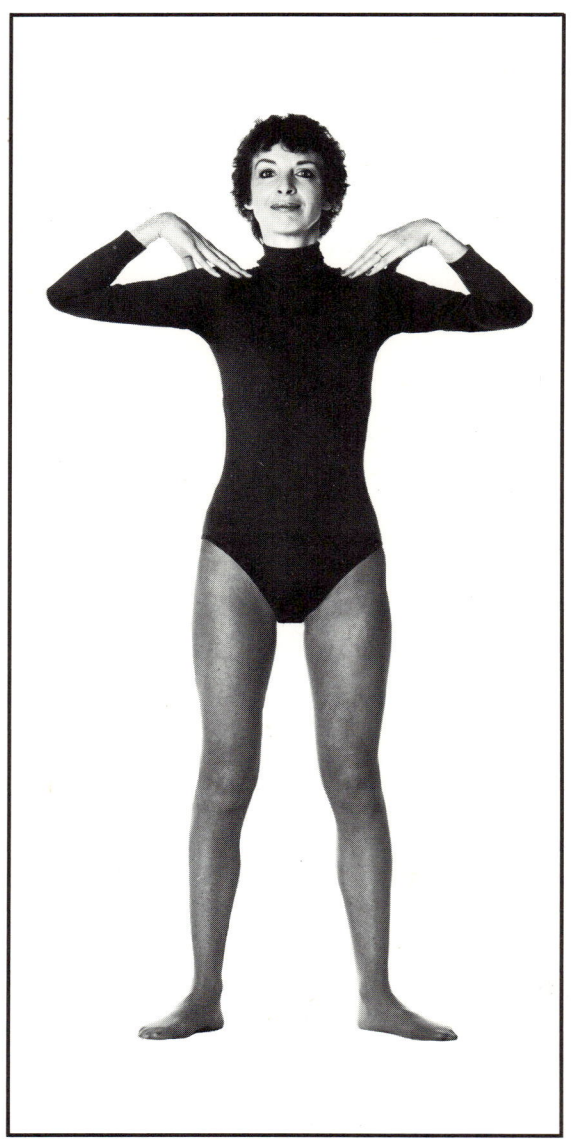

THE SHOULDERS

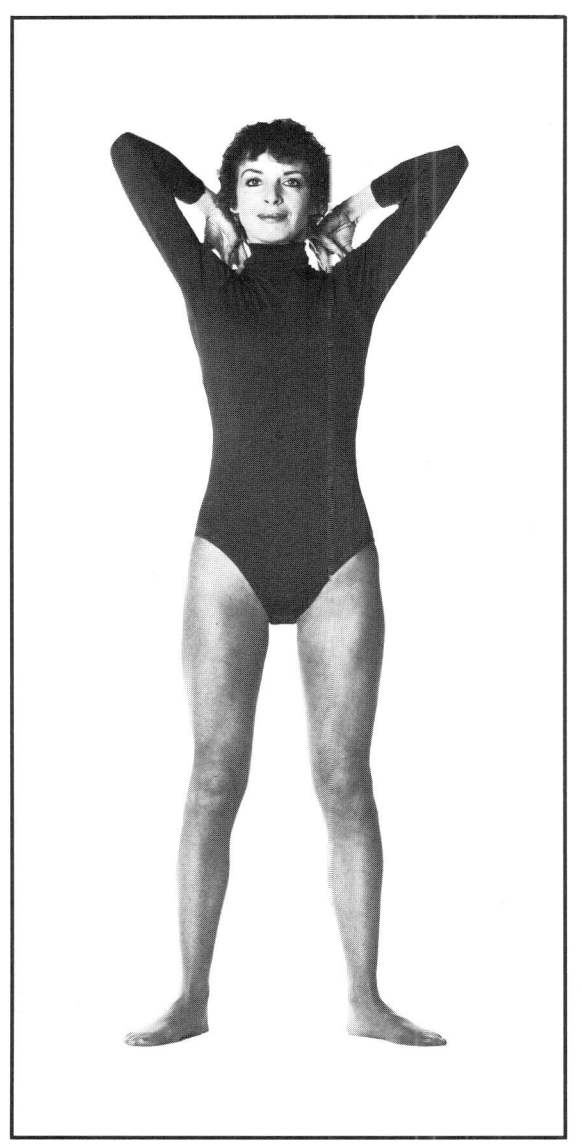 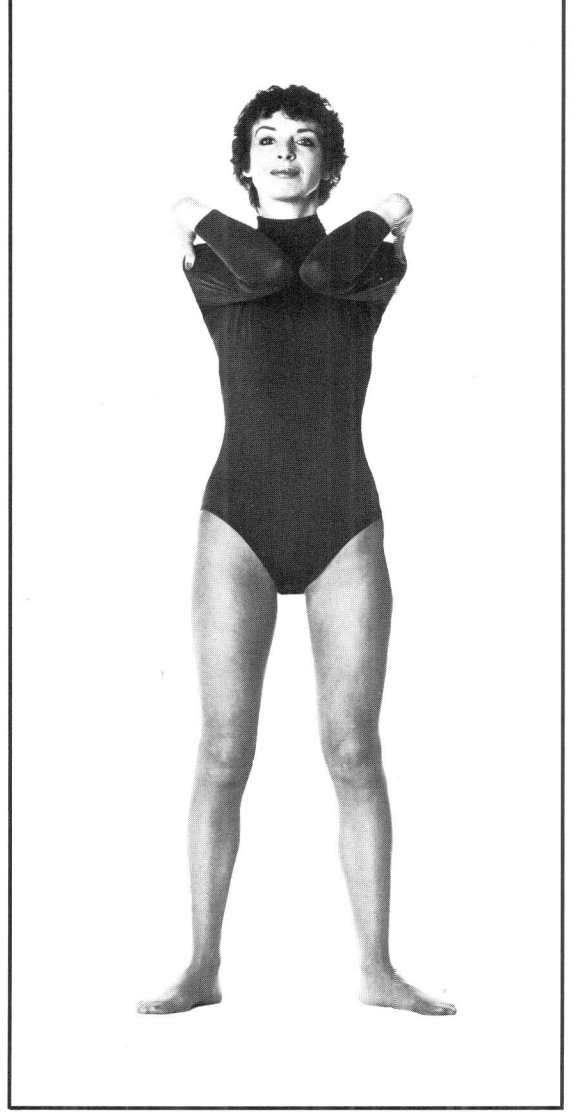

THE SHOULDERS III

1.* Place your hands on your shoulders so that your elbows are out at either side of you. Now just keep pumping your elbows back. Push and pump. You should really feel your shoulder blades being squeezed together.

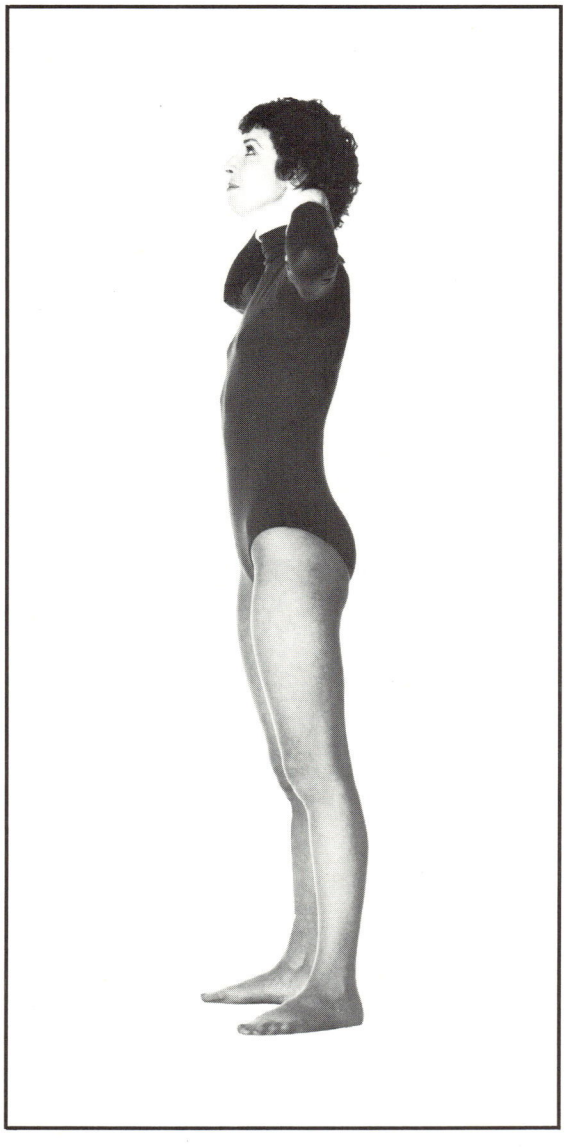

THE SHOULDERS 39

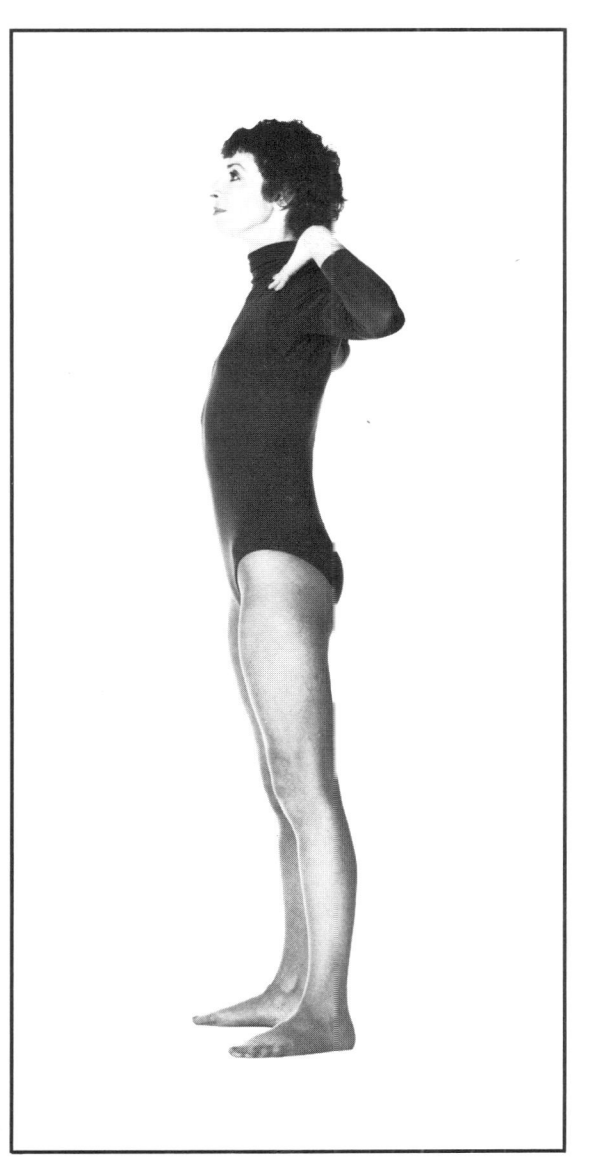

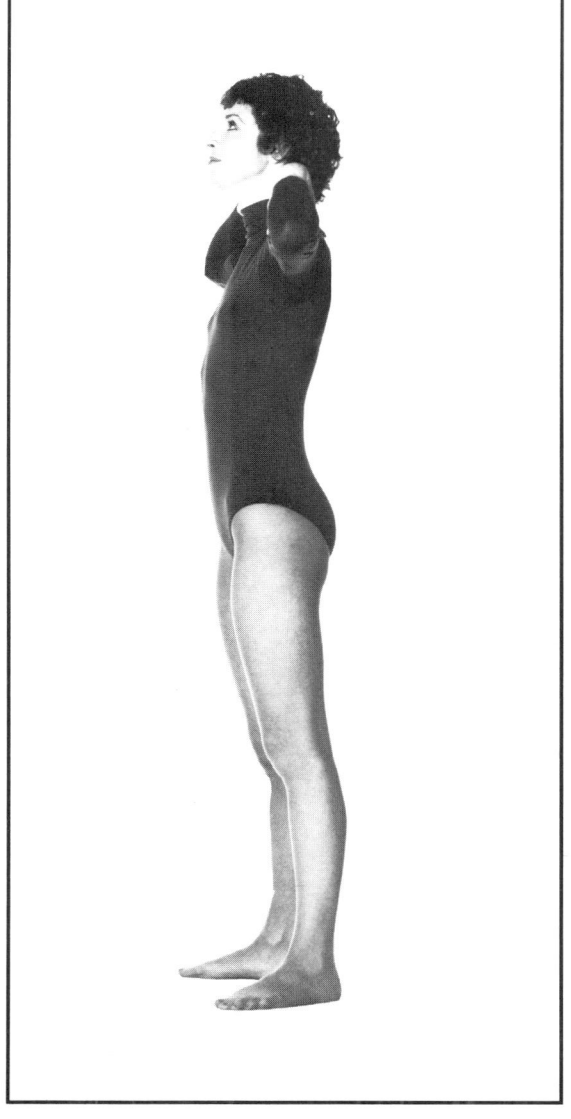

THE SHOULDERS IV

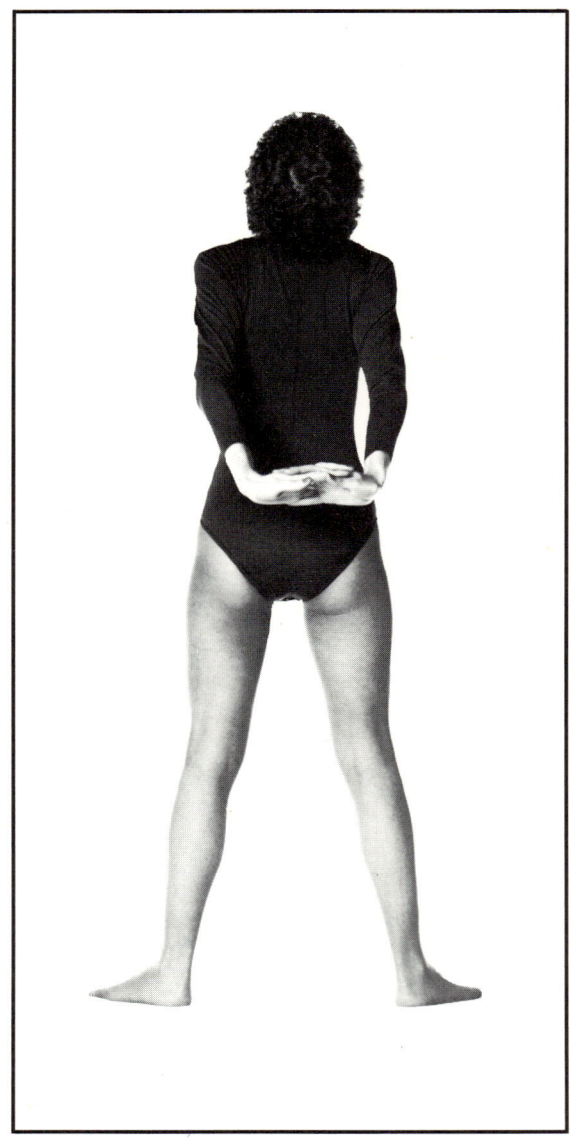

This exercise is a great help towards better posture. If you're one of those people who slump when they sit, or on seeing your reflection in the mirror are horrified at the hunchback you're developing, then this is certainly the exercise for you! It's also good for children who tend to be casual slumpers.

Do this exercise morning and evening.

1.** Stand very straight and tall. Clasp your hands together behind you interlocking your fingers. Turn your hands inside out so that your palms are facing outwards. Push back your shoulder blades and face the ceiling.

Now pump your clasped hands upwards at least five times. Gradually increase the number of times you do this, and you will become less round-shouldered and loosen your tensions. The more you do this exercise the easier it becomes.

THE SHOULDERS 41

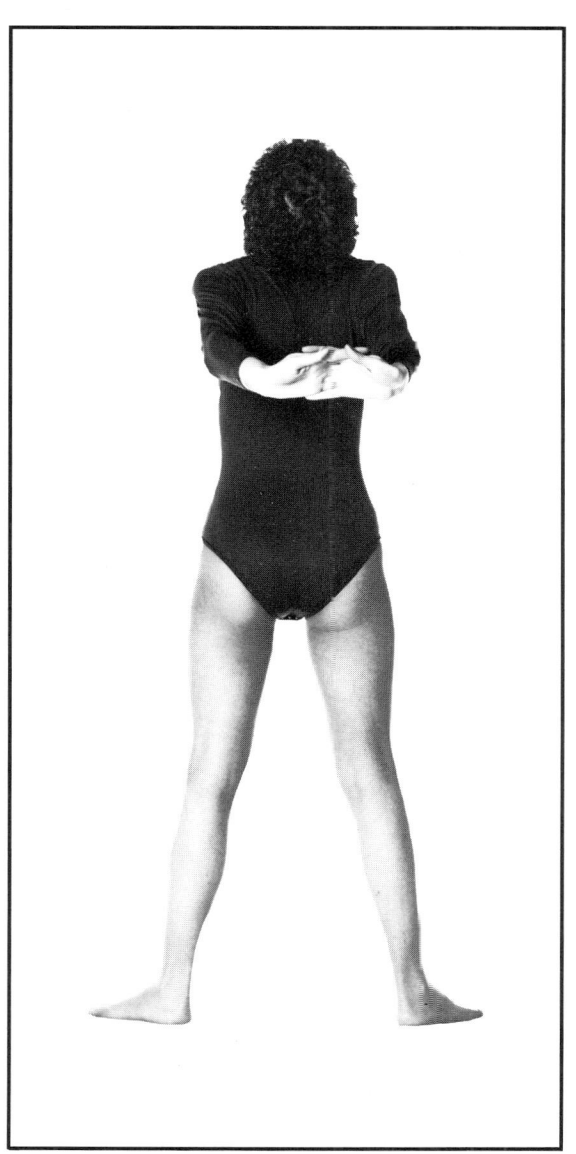
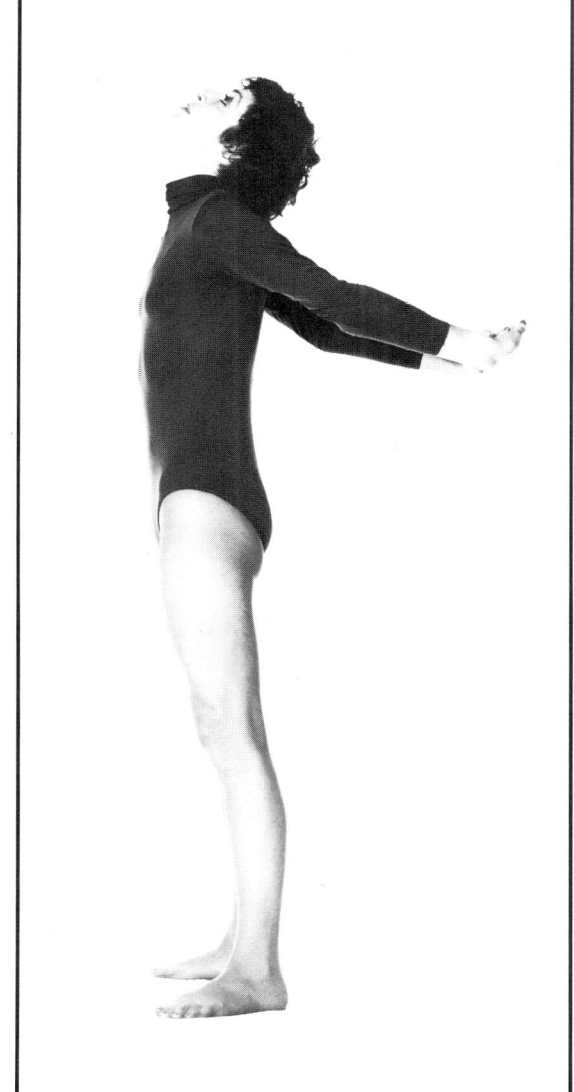

THE SHOULDERS
V

These exercises not only strengthen your shoulders, but are good for various other parts of the body as well. They utilize the pectoral muscle, thereby helping to tone up your bosoms; they increase the flexibility of your spine; and they help greatly to strengthen your wrists—vital for those of us who have to screw tops off recalcitrant jars, or wring out clothes.

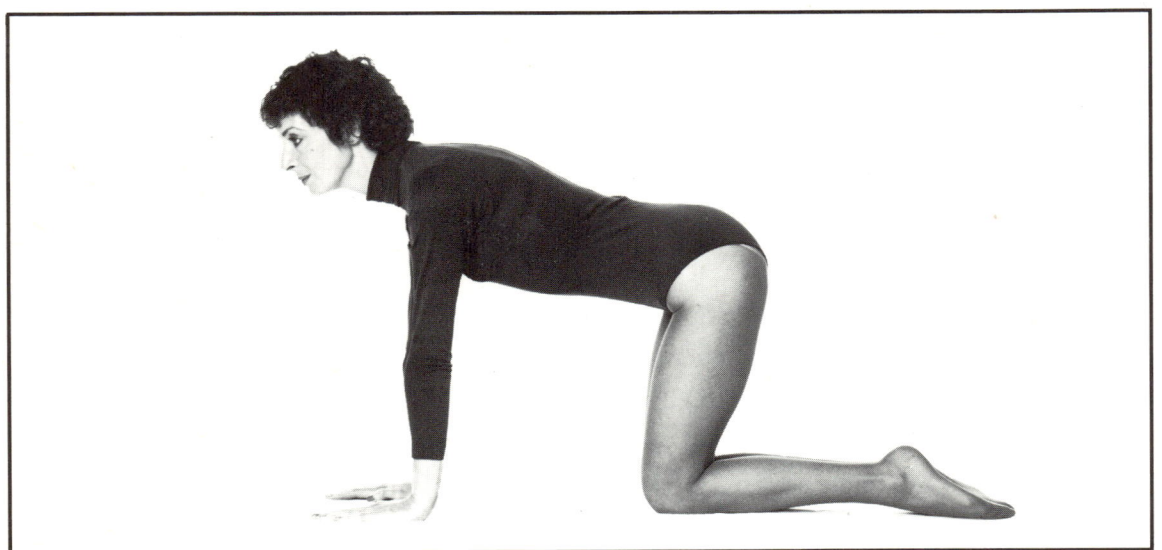

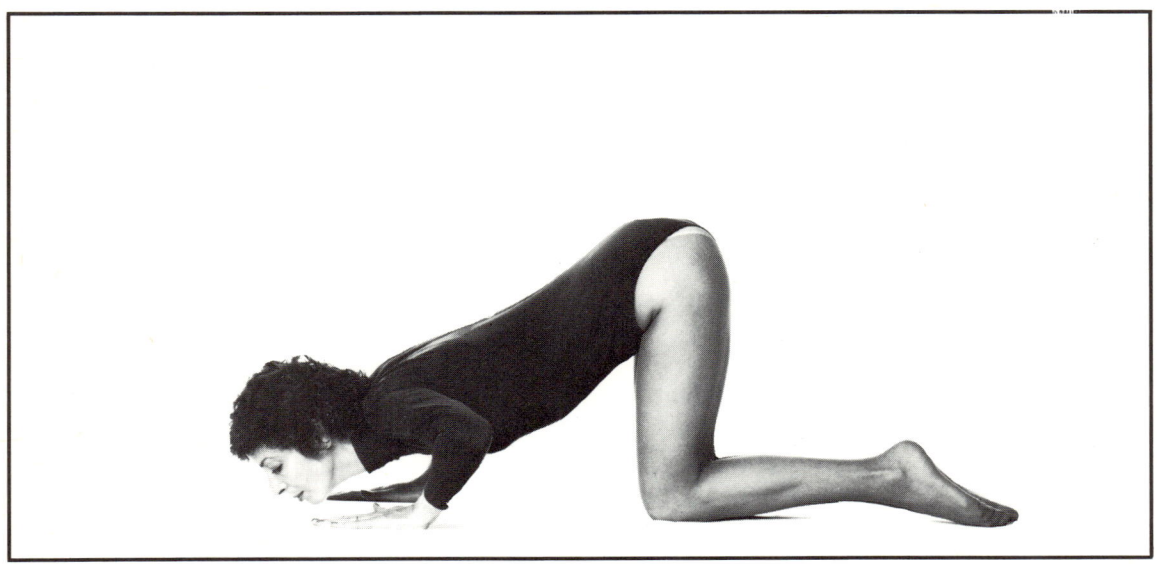

1.* Get down on the floor on all fours. Bend your arms, elbows up, and bring your chin down to the floor. Do this movement at least five times.

2.** Still on all fours, lift one leg up high and outstretched. Stretch your arms to a locked position and bend them again until your chin touches the floor. Repeat five times then change to the other leg.

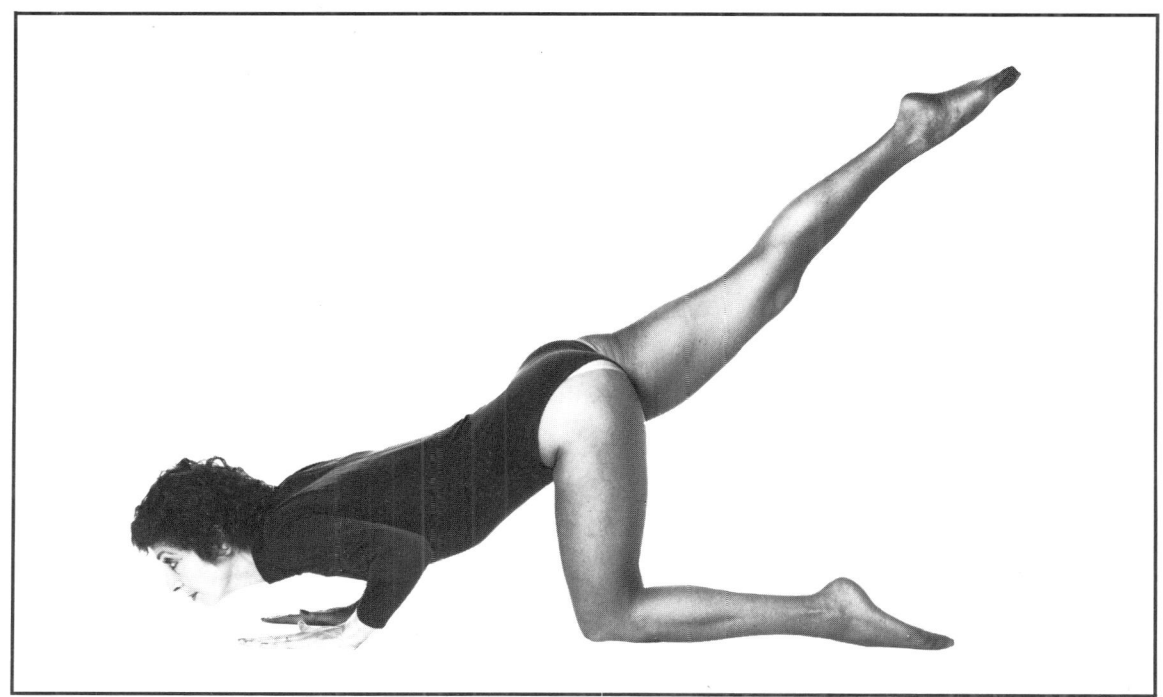

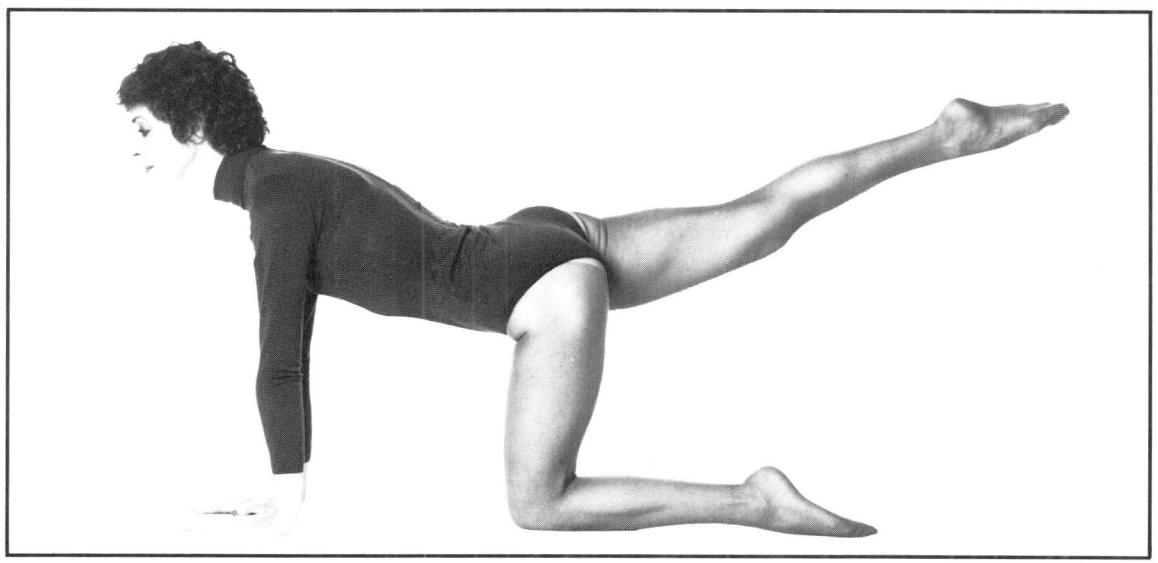

THE BACK

Backache is almost more common than the common cold. It causes more discomfort and pain, and therefore more weeks off work, than any other illness. One of the causes of backache over which we have little or no control is the fact that man's physical evolution has been slower than his cerebral. Structurally we are still more of a four-legged animal forced by our needs and way of life over the years to stand upright. Our spine and pelvis have not as yet attained equal development in the evolutionary process with that of our brains.

But basically most back problems are due to bad posture, lifting things incorrectly, carrying objects without distributing the weight evenly and so on. Even the way you carry your handbag can have an effect on your back. For instance it is better to carry your handbag in your hand straight down at your side, or better still wear a shoulderstrap; *don't* carry it over a bent arm. Naturally this also applies to your shopping. Carry it properly.

Walking and lying down are really the safest activities for your back, and even when lying down, you should be sure it's a good firm surface that will support your body with no sag. To test this, place a full cup of tea on your bed and then sit on the bed. If some tea spills into the saucer your bed is too soft. This can easily be rectified by slipping a wooden board between the base and the mattress (and saves the price of a new bed!).

THE BACK I

Every time you do an exercise involving the muscles in your back, you should finish off with this relaxing exercise.

1. Kneel with your hands on the floor so that you're on all fours like a dog. Arch your spine placing your head down so that your chin presses towards your chest and your tail is tucked in.

Reverse now so that you hollow your back bringing your head up and sticking your bottom out. Do this slowly and gently as often as you like.

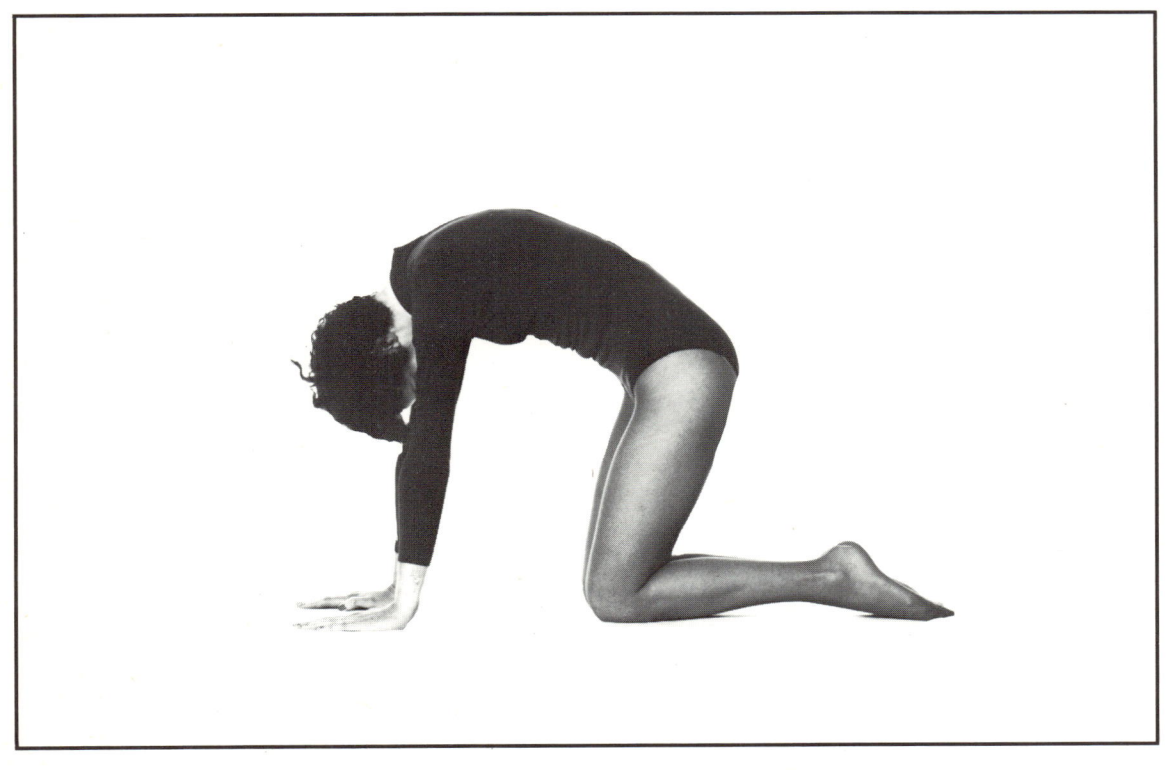

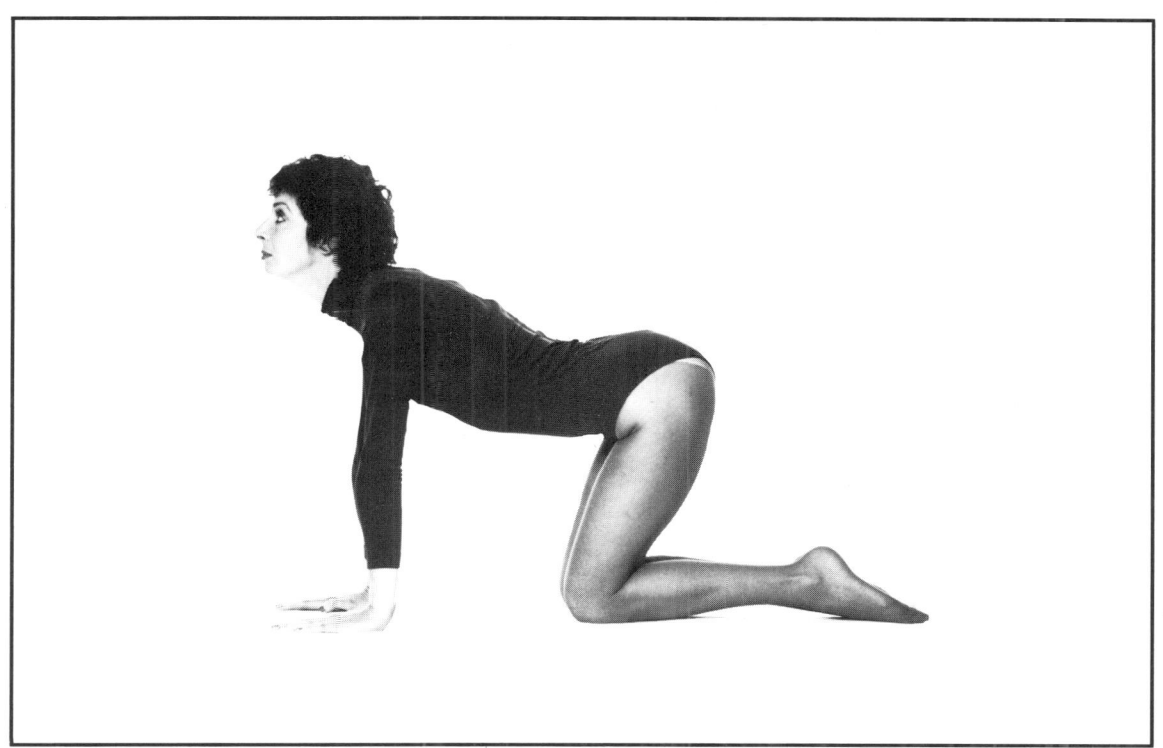

THE BACK II

Heavy manual labour, pregnancy, sitting for long periods at a desk job or long car journeys (car seats are one of the most acute causes of backache): these are just a few of the many pressures we put on the spine and pelvis. The following exercises should help strengthen your back muscles and to some degree alleviate backache.

1.** Take a small flattish cushion to give yourself a little comfort while doing this exercise. Lie flat on the floor face down. Place the cushion under your pelvis. Put your hands on the floor beside your bottom. Now gently and slowly raise your head and shoulders off the ground keeping your feet and legs on the floor. Hold it to the count of five. Relax.

2.* This time as you lift your head and shoulders off the floor, put your hands on your bottom and raise your legs as well. Hold it to the count of five. Relax.

This exercise should be done gently and slowly. Don't pull up jerkily or pull up too high. Remember to keep your head, shoulders and legs just off the floor.

3. Finish off with the Back Relaxer Exercise, page 46.

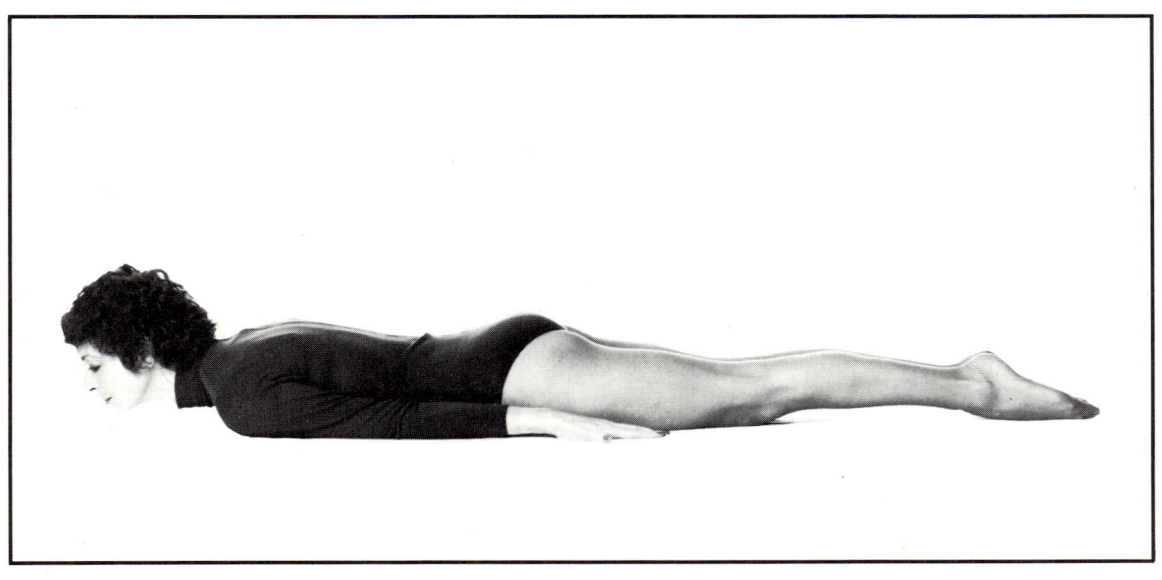

THE BACK 49

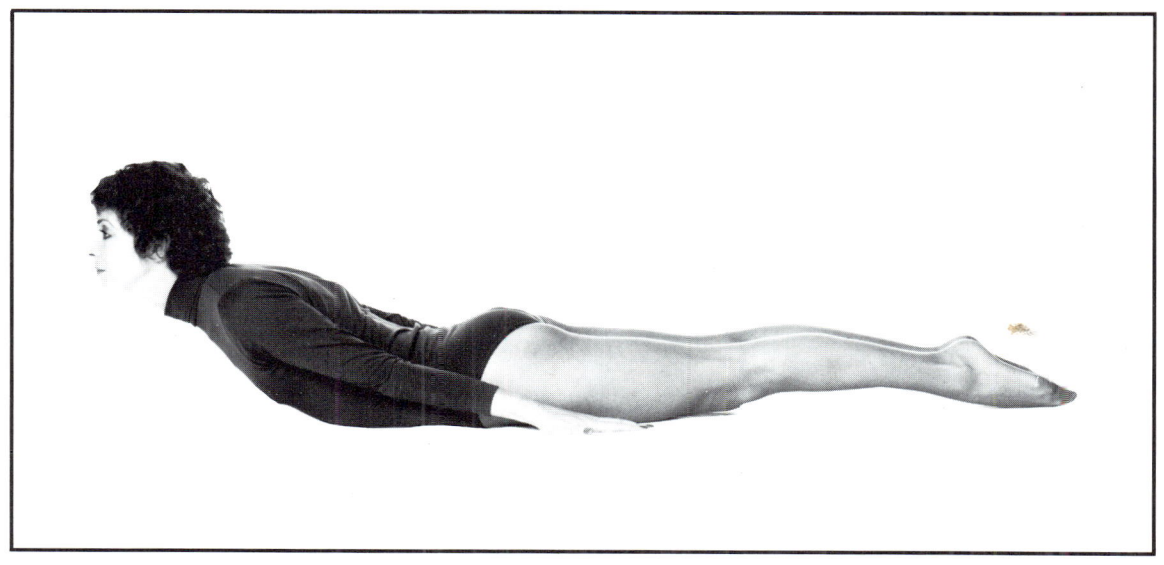

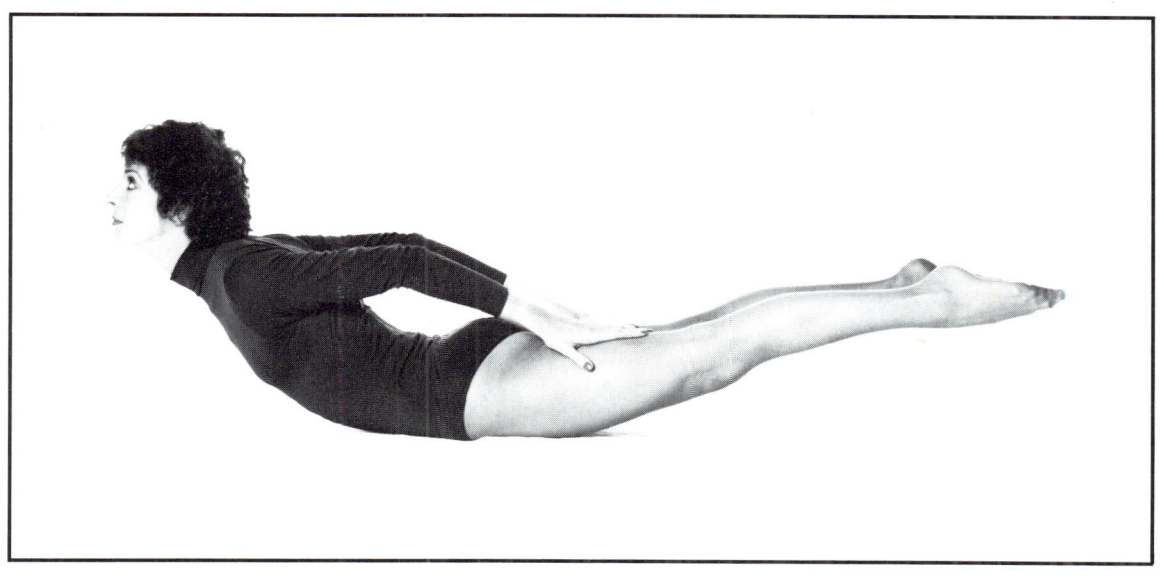

THE BACK III

Lie on the floor face down with a small flattish cushion under your pelvis. Keep your legs together and nicely stretched. Keep your legs on the floor throughout this exercise.

1.** Stretch your arms out in front of you and start doing the breast stroke.

As your arms come round to your sides and back you lift your head and shoulders off the floor.

As you bring your arms together and back to your original position, lower your head and shoulders so that you are ready to begin again. You should keep a nice and gentle breast stroke going without any stops and starts. Try for five to start with and aim for ten.

2. Finish off with the Back Relaxer Exercise, page 46.

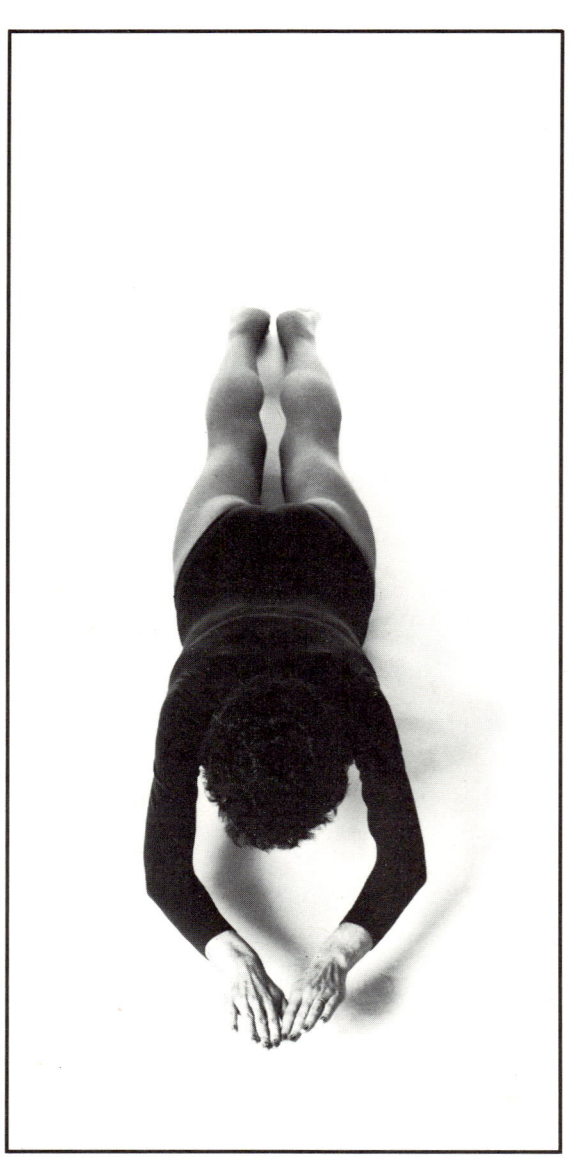

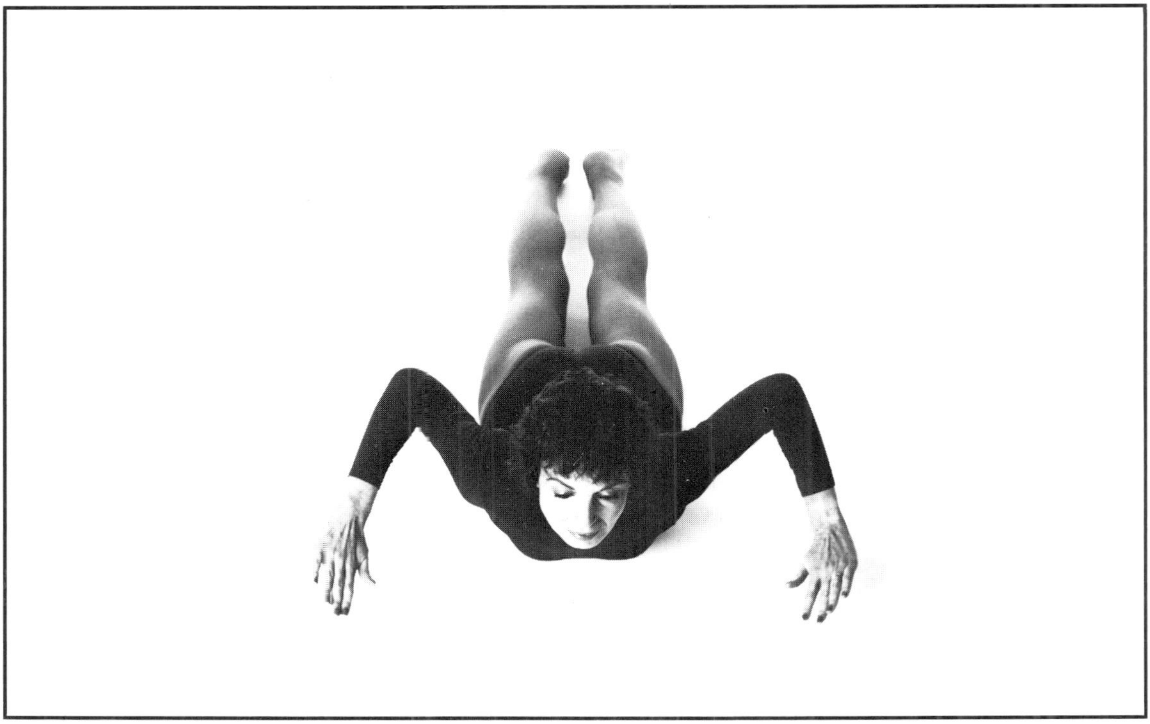

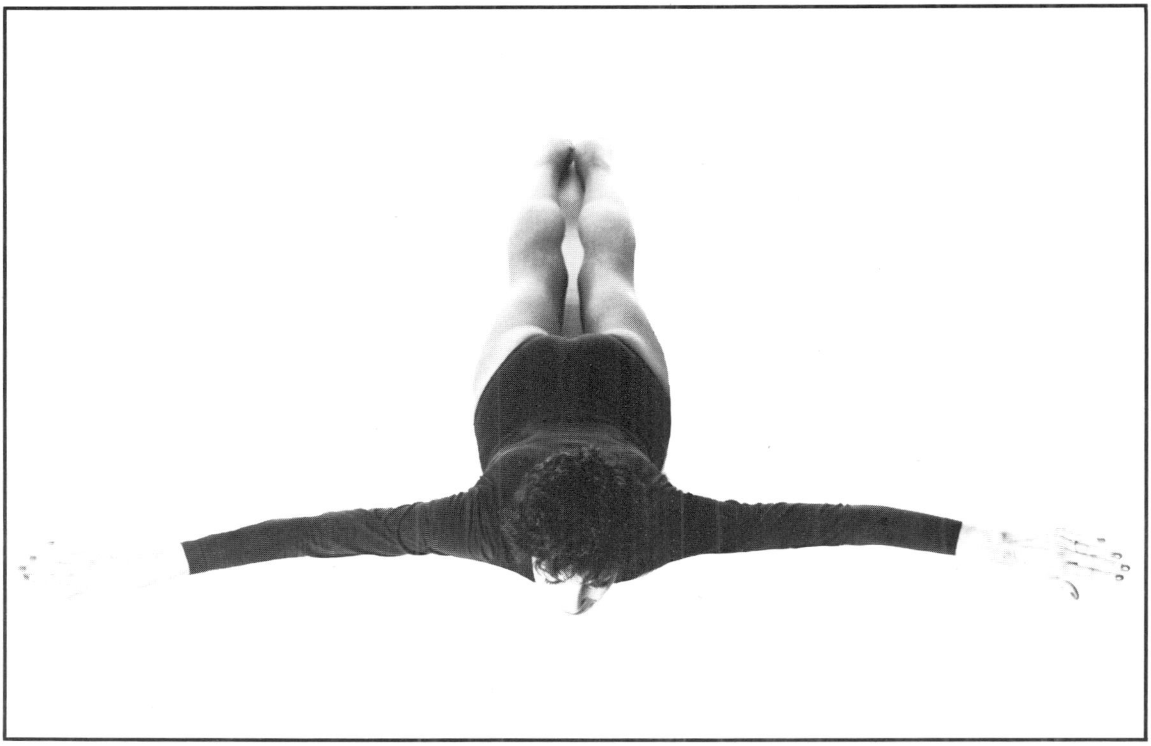

THE BACK 51

THE BACK IV

This exercise will give your spine an excellent stretch, and strengthen all the muscles in your back.

1.* Kneel on all fours.

Raise one leg and stretch it out behind you.

Lift up the opposite arm to the leg that is raised and stretch your arm out in front of you. Hold this position for the count of ten.

Return to the original position and repeat the exercise with your other leg and arm.

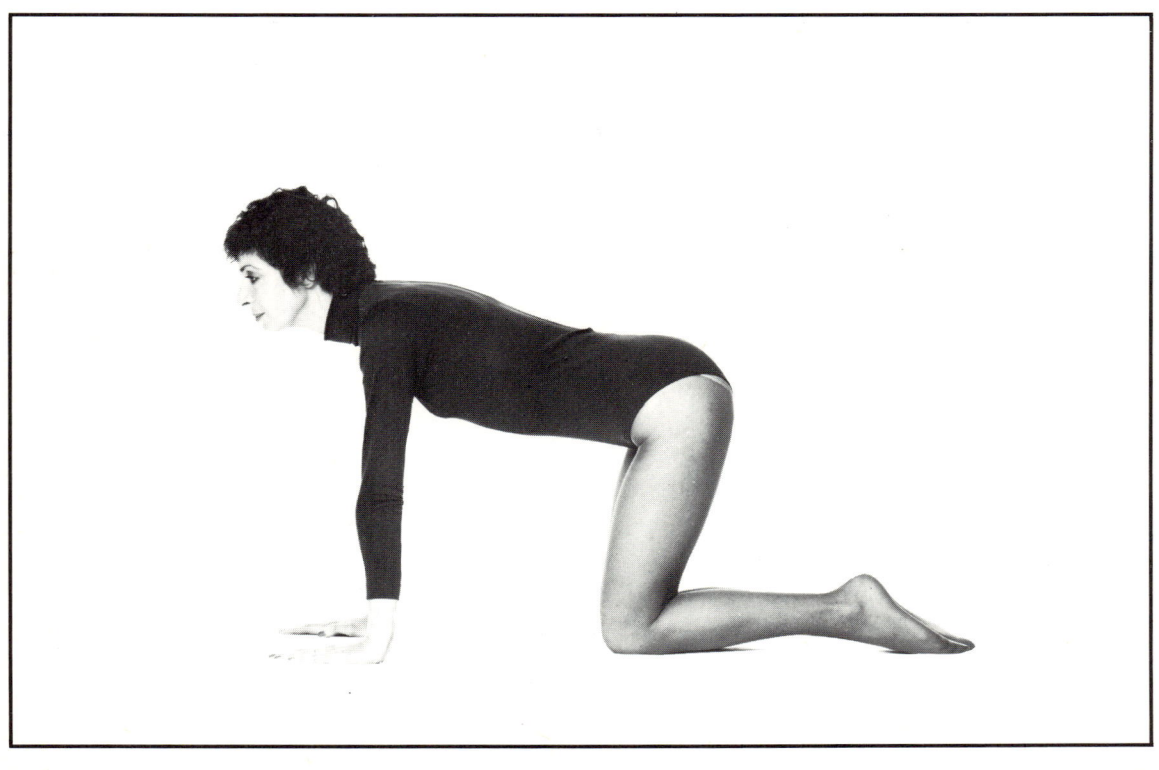

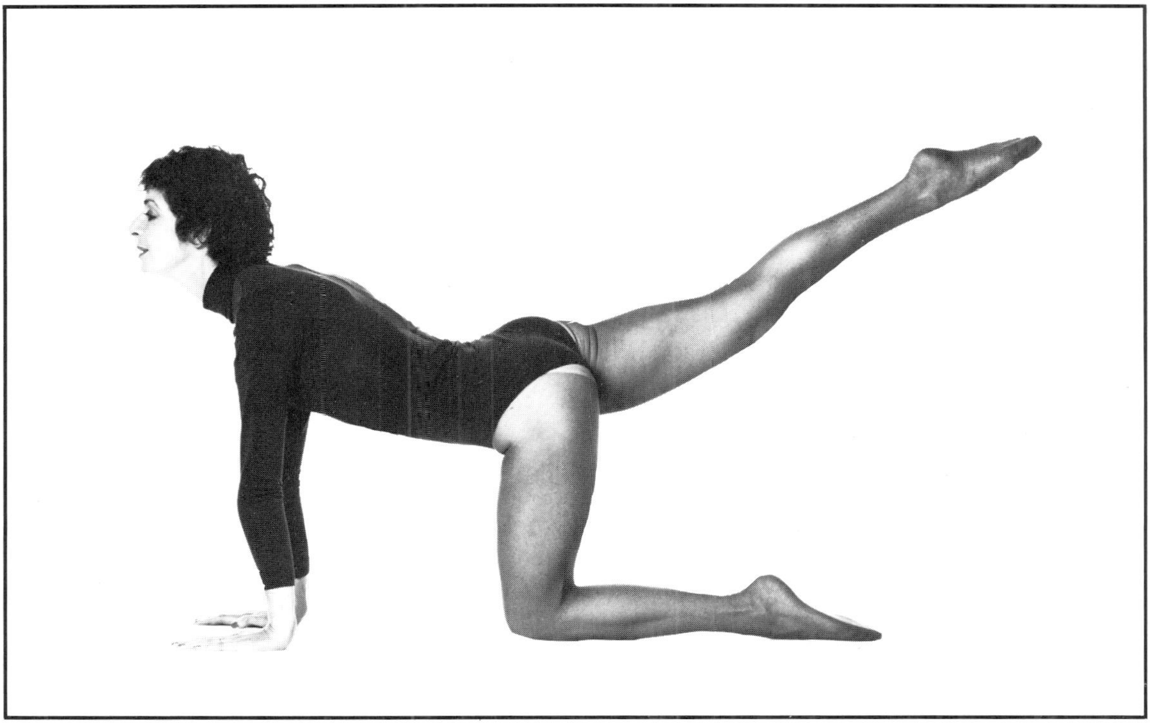

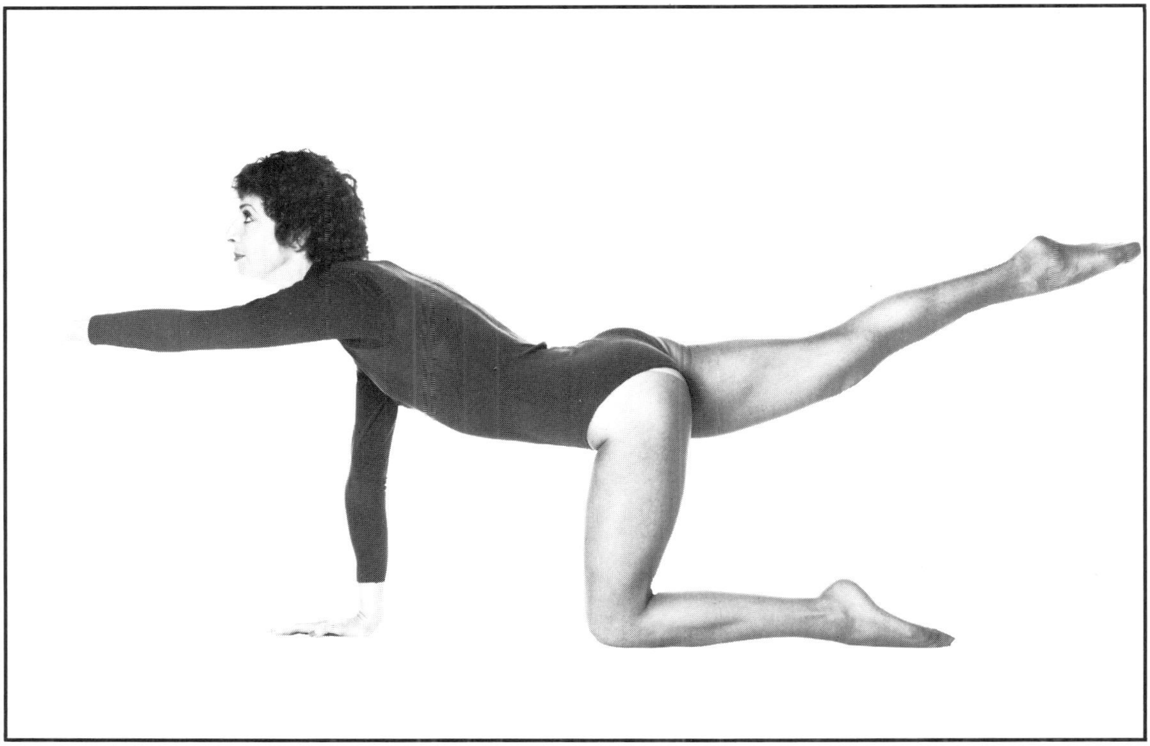

THE BACK 53

THE STOMACH

The waistline is not only the first place to become flabby, but also the first place to be seen to be flabby. The flab may begin by seeming no worse than a bicycle tyre. If possible, you shouldn't even allow this stage to be reached because in no time at all your spare tyre could develop into a car tyre, and then you have problems.

Your eating habits are mostly responsible for this spare tyre. I can't stress enough how important it is to watch your health by watching your weight; you must eat the right foods—*whole* foods. Keep away from refined and processed foods and away from crash or faddy diets. You should be able to lose unwanted pounds without the use of a diet (most diets, after all, are temporary, and you could easily revert to your old eating habits—the ones that caused the weight in the first place).

Between your rib cage and your pelvis, only one thing is keeping you upright besides your muscles, and that is your spine. If you think of the large proportion of body your spine is having to hold upright, you can easily understand the importance of building up the strength of your abdominal muscles. If you don't exercise these muscles regularly, you add an unnecessary burden to your spine which can cause backache: many of the stomach exercises in the pages following are specifically designed to restore resilience to neglected muscles and thereby help prevent backache. Not exercising these muscles also allows you too easily to fall victim to that dreaded spare tyre. So you see it makes sense to work at the exercises and aim for a trim waist-line, not simply for a better and more shapely appearance, but for better health.

THE STOMACH I

1.* Sit on the floor on a flattish cushion. Bend your knees keeping your feet firmly on the ground. Place your hands on your knees. Keep your back very straight.

Now squeeze your buttocks together and curl your spine from your hips only, so that your vertebrae are gently, in turn, pressed down on the floor. Don't try to go too low at first. If you can lower the upper half of you so that your arms are stretched this is an excellent beginning. By always being sure that the vertebrae of your lumbar region are pressed firmly into the floor you will use all your stomach muscles which will become firmer more quickly and not put any strain on your back. Sit up straight again and practise the buttock squeezing movement.

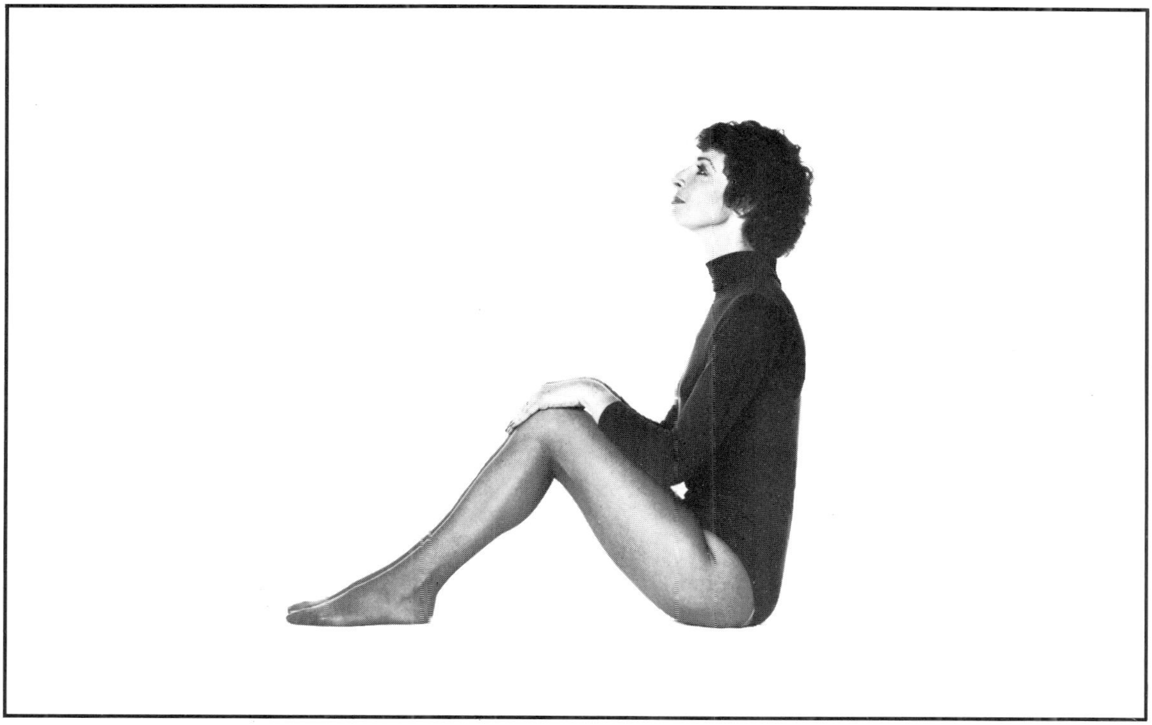

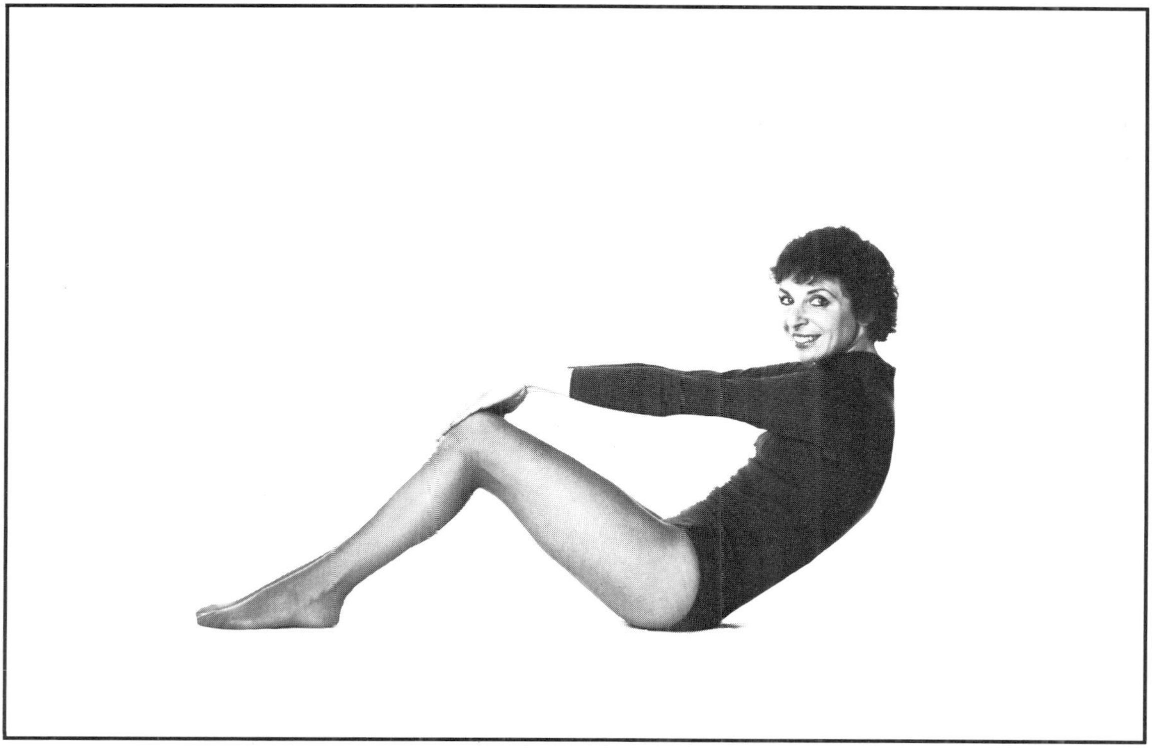

THE STOMACH 57

THE STOMACH II

1.** Sit on the floor, hands on your knees, as in the previous exercise. Squeeze your buttocks together and curl your spine until your arms are outstretched, your hands still on your knees.

Raise one arm up as close to your head as possible keeping it straight. Place it back on your knee, and raise your other arm up. Try for five arm lifts with each arm.

I cannot stress enough the importance of the position of your lower back. It should be kept curled and pressed into the floor for maximum effect.

2.** Raise both hands off your knees as high as is comfortable without losing your position. Place hands back on knees. Try this five times and increase as you become stronger.

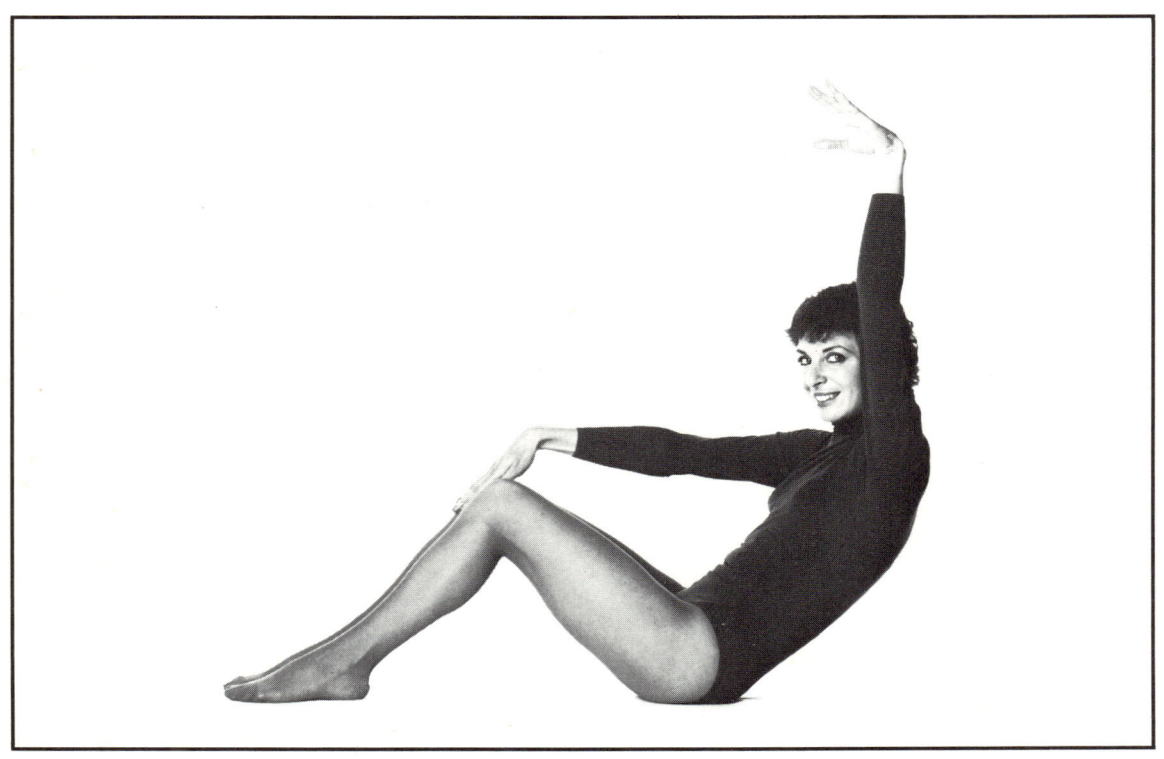

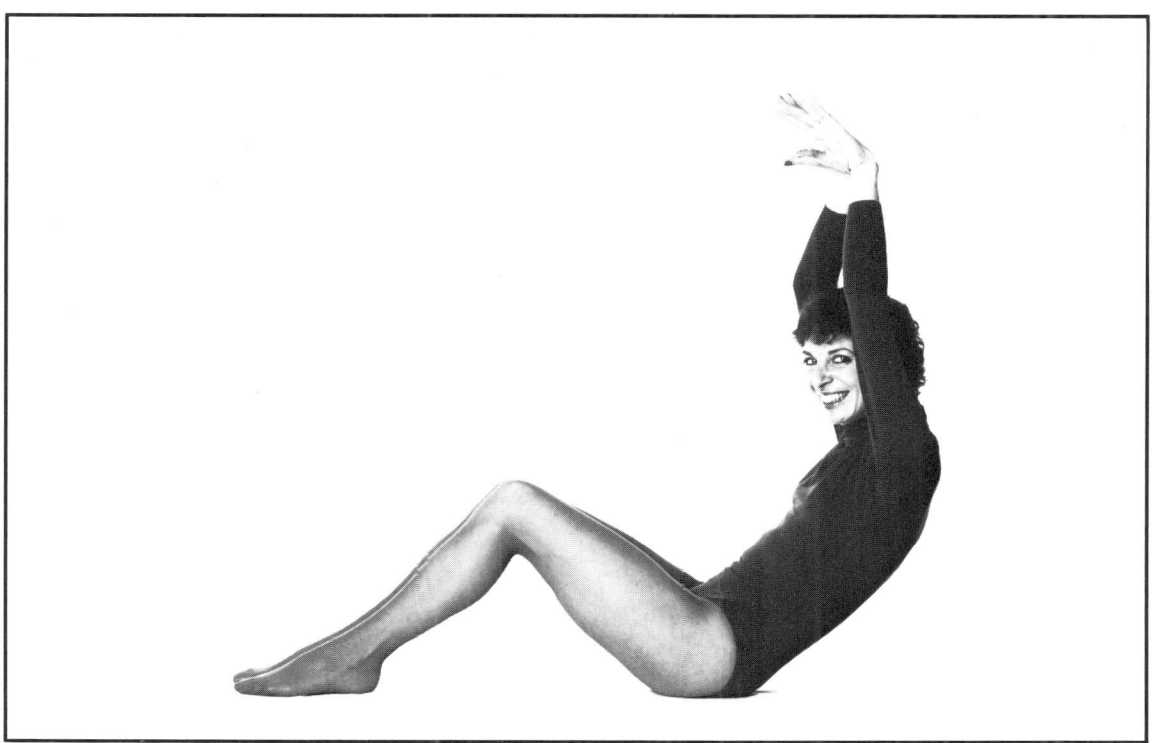

THE STOMACH III

1.** Lie flat on your back with your arms down by your sides. Squeeze your buttocks together so that the small of your back is pressed firmly into the floor.

Raise one leg up so that your foot is pointing to the ceiling. Now lift the other leg one inch off the floor. Check that you are still in position. The small of your back must be pressed into the floor at all times during this exercise.

Now 'walk'. Make big strides and get a nice easy walking motion. Never let the lower leg touch the floor, just allow it to come down to within an inch or two of the floor. Keep your legs stretched tautly with nicely pointed toes.

2.*** If you can, raise your head off the floor and look at your toes. This will make your stomach muscles work even harder. And if you can after a while (maybe several sessions) raise the upper part of your shoulders off the floor you will be making splendid progress and should already be noticing that slack muscles are really firming up and giving you shape.

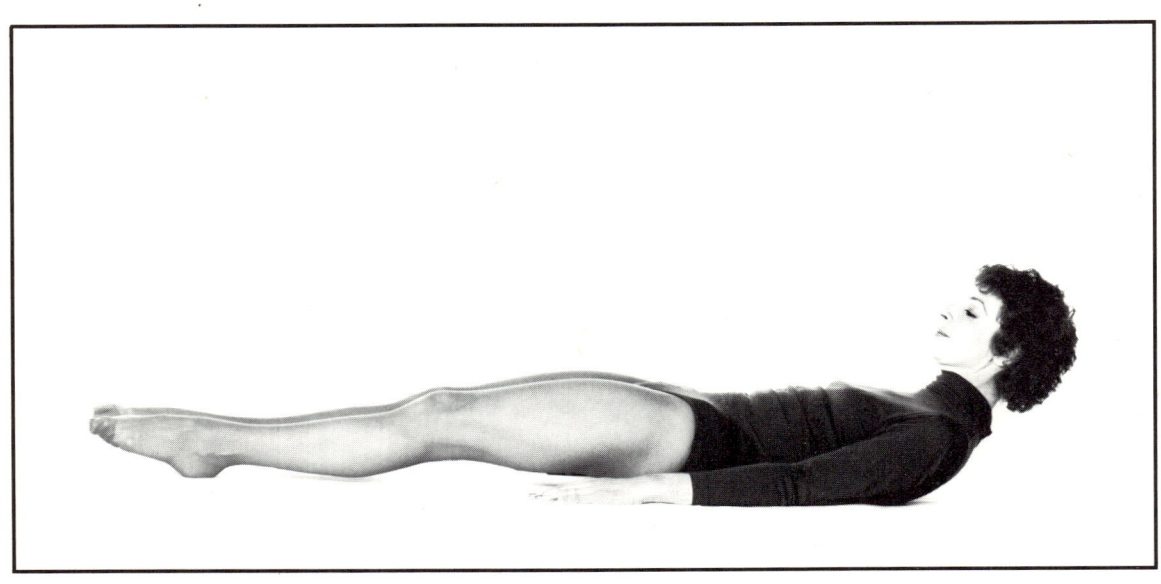

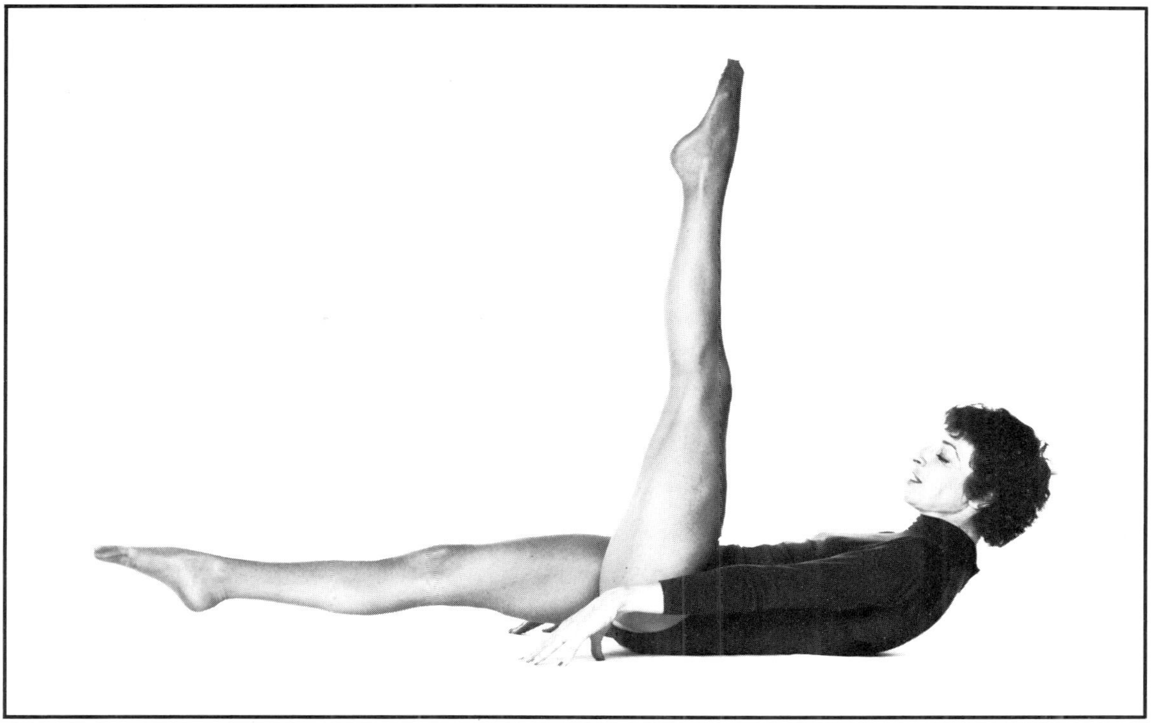

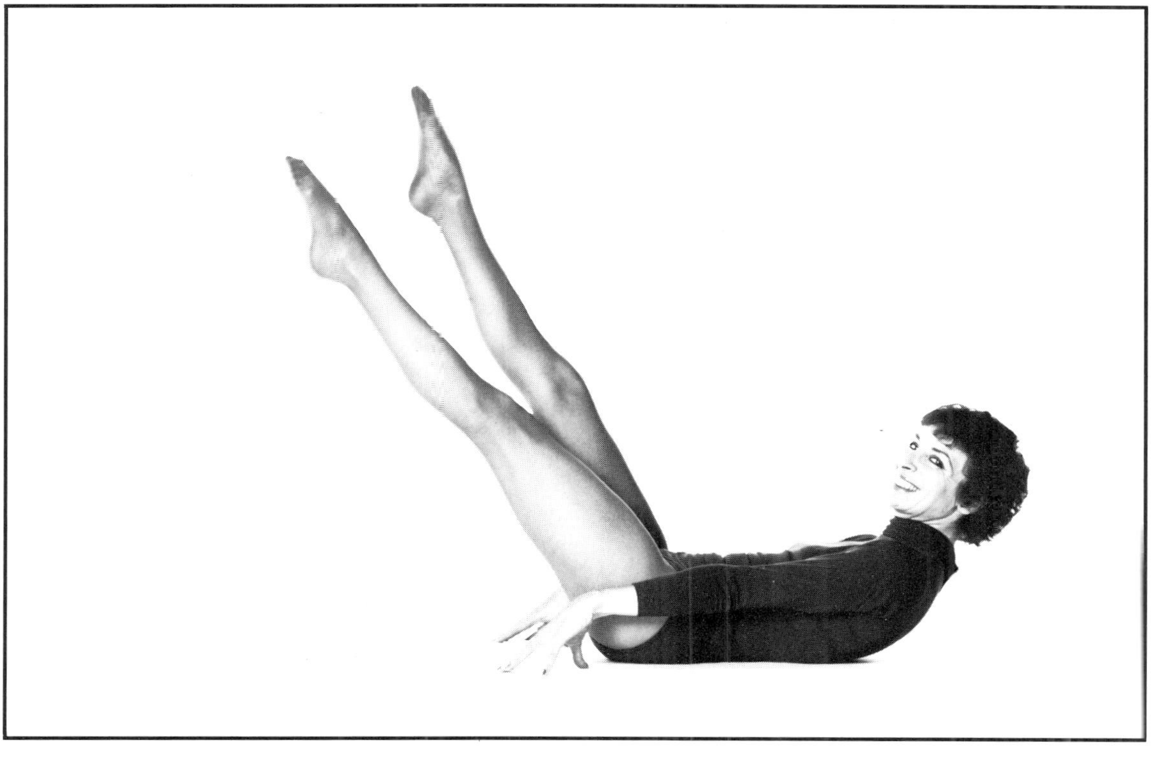

THE STOMACH

THE STOMACH IV

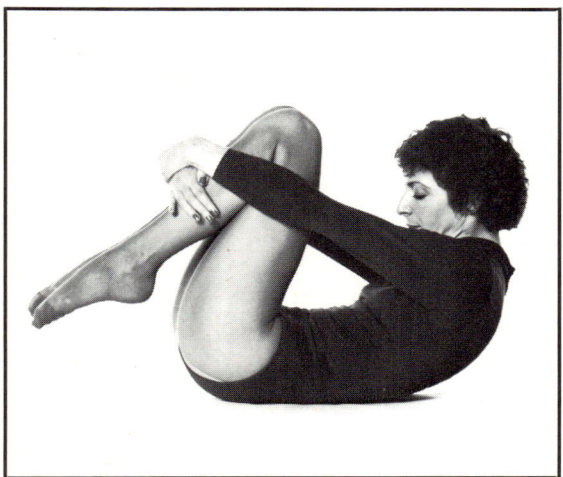

1.*** Lie on your back on the floor. Curl up into a ball so that your knees are bent close to your chest, your head raised off the floor and curled down onto your chest as close to your knees as you can. Place your arms round your knees. You should now be completely curled round.

Take your arms away.

Stretch your legs straight up towards the ceiling and stretch your fingers up towards your toes. Still keep your chin tucked well down on your chest. And try to keep the upper part of your shoulders rounded off the floor.

Slowly lower one leg down and allow it to lightly touch the floor. Don't let it bang down and relax, as this will throw your body out of its original and important position. Raise the leg up again until it is parallel with your other leg. Lower the other leg. Once you have stretched your legs keep them beautifully stretched right through to your toes so you feel like a ballet dancer. Really point your toes and keep your knees locked. Repeat this. One up, one down, several times.

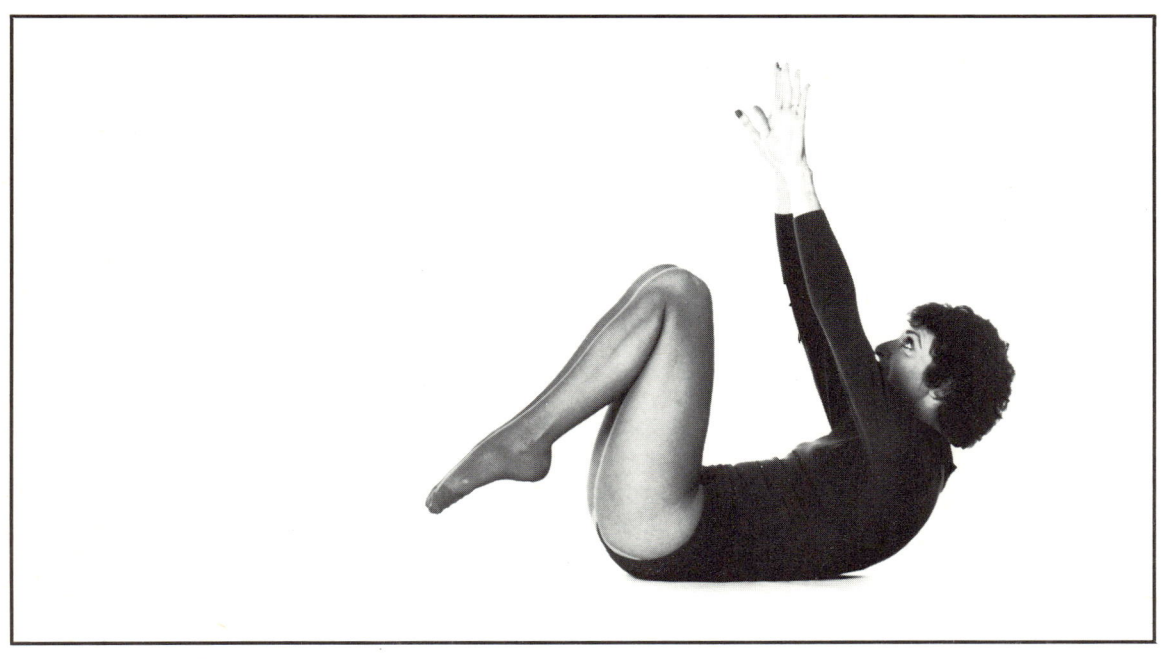

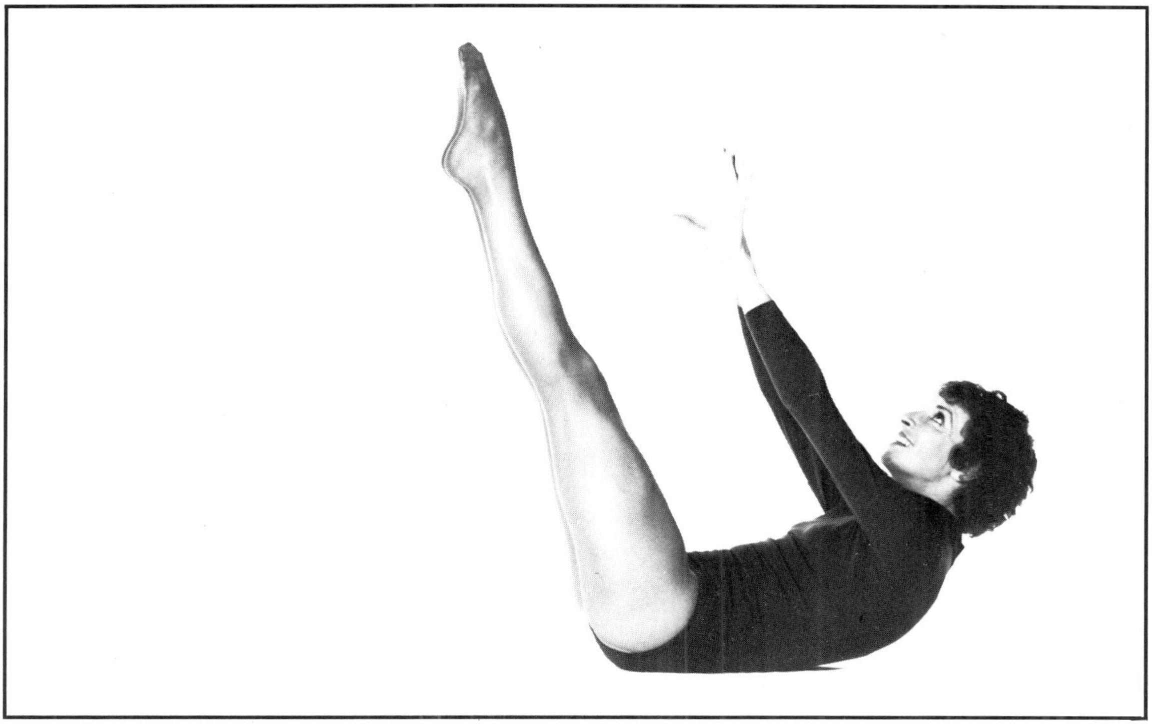

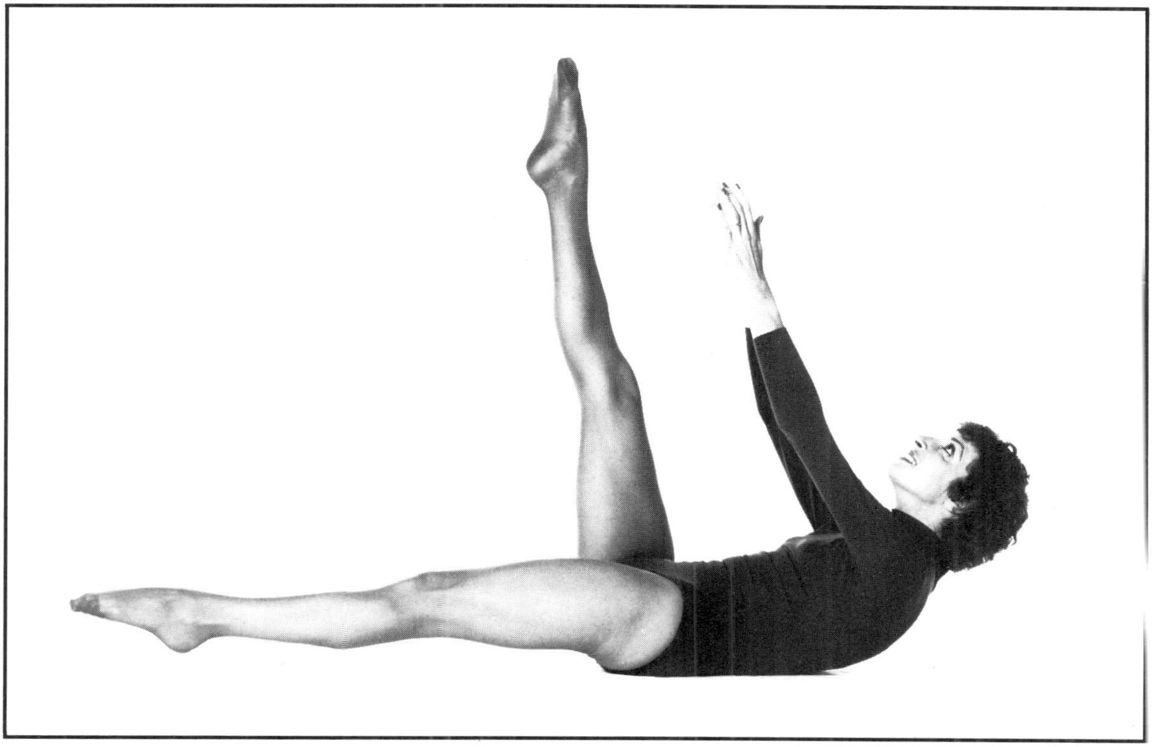

THE STOMACH 33

THE STOMACH V

This particular exercise concentrates on your muscles from the waist up. So while you exercise your waist you also exercise the muscles all around your rib cage and abdomen.

All the stomach exercises require effort, but it is really worth while getting this one right. The results give an excellent shape and outline to your figure.

You will need a kitchen chair (an armchair isn't suitable as the seat is usually too low) which is of the right height to make the exercise effective—although difficult.

1.***** Lie on your back and place your feet and calves on the chair seat.

Now, using your arms to help you, swing upwards so that your head and shoulders come off the floor. It is important to aim to get your shoulder blades off the floor. Try for five swings at first, working up with practise, to at least twenty.

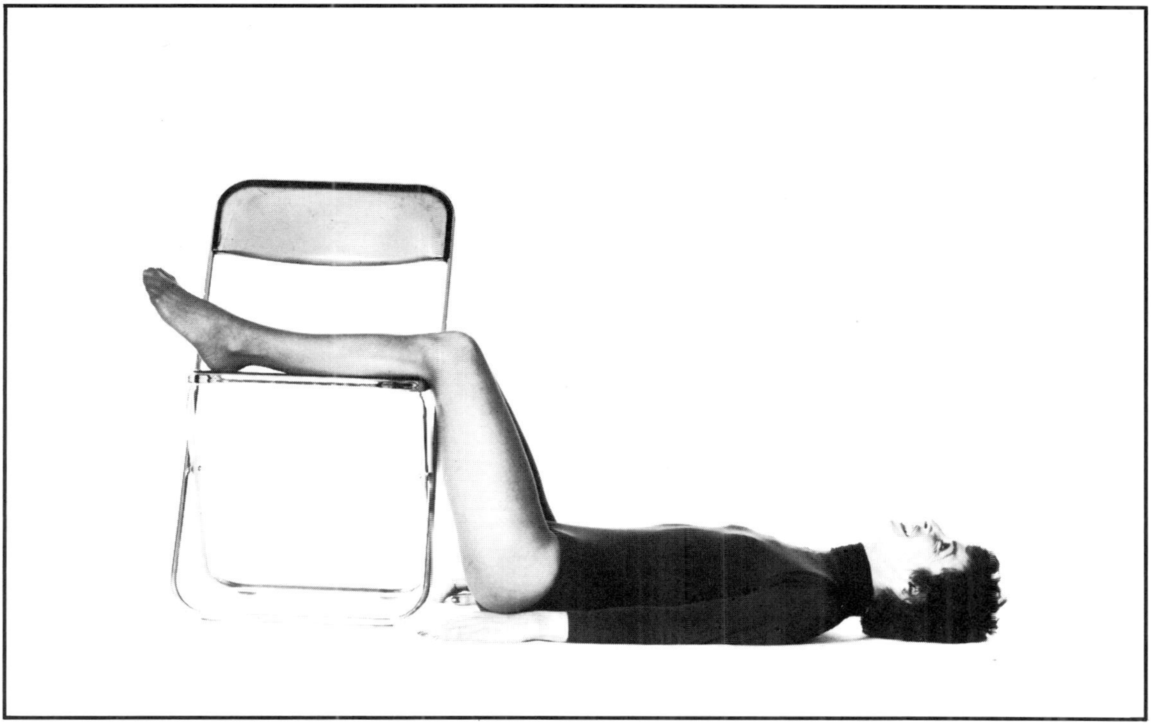

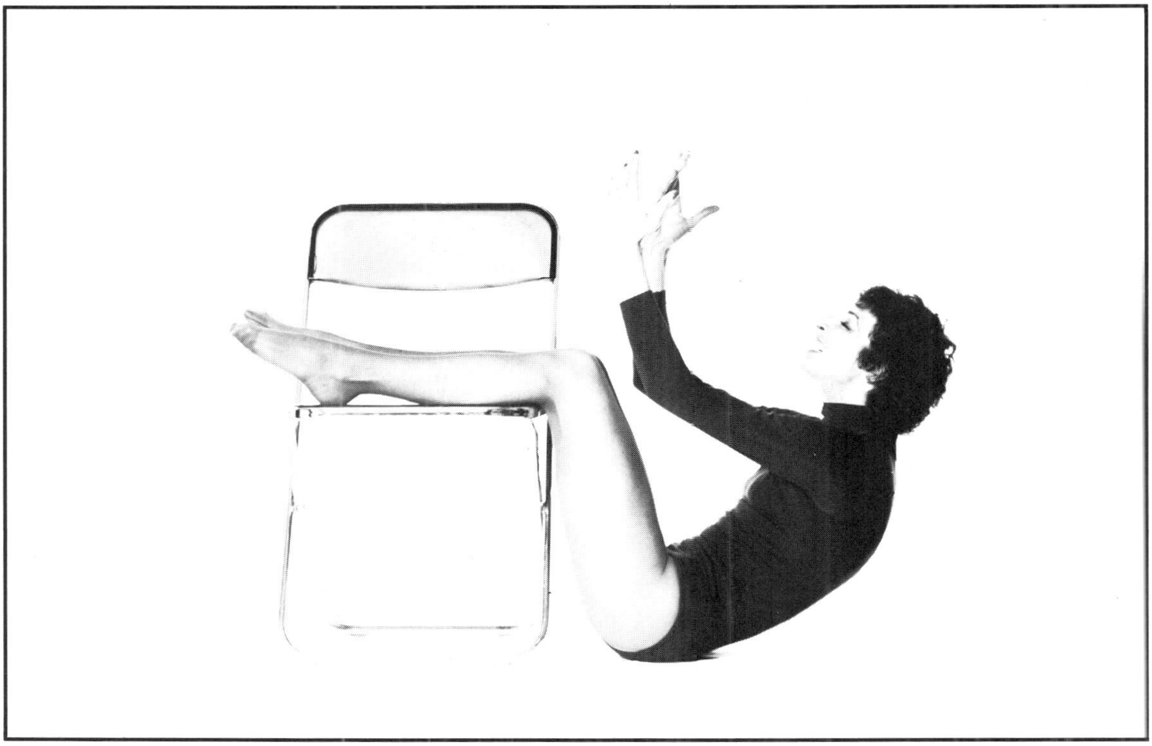

THE STOMACH 65

THE STOMACH & THIGHS

Individually, the stomach and the thighs are two of the classic problem areas, so I make no excuses for offering a separate section which includes both together. Both areas suffer from all the faults common to other problem areas: lack of muscle control and overeating.

If you don't want to be corseted, you must have *natural* control, which means exercising your stomach muscles. The thigh muscles too, don't get used enough, which is why so many of us, men and women alike, get flabby there. If you consciously hold in your stomach muscles all the time, and pull up your buttock and thigh muscles when you sit for instance, it can quickly become a habit and help enormously. But there is nothing to beat exercises, and there is a great variety in the pages following from which to choose.

THE STOMACH & THIGHS I

This is a marvellous exercise for pulling up and firming the lower abdominal muscles.

1.★ Sit on the floor. Place your hands on the floor either side of your bottom for support.

Bend one leg and keep the foot on the floor. Stretch the other leg out in front of you with a nicely pointed toe. Raise your

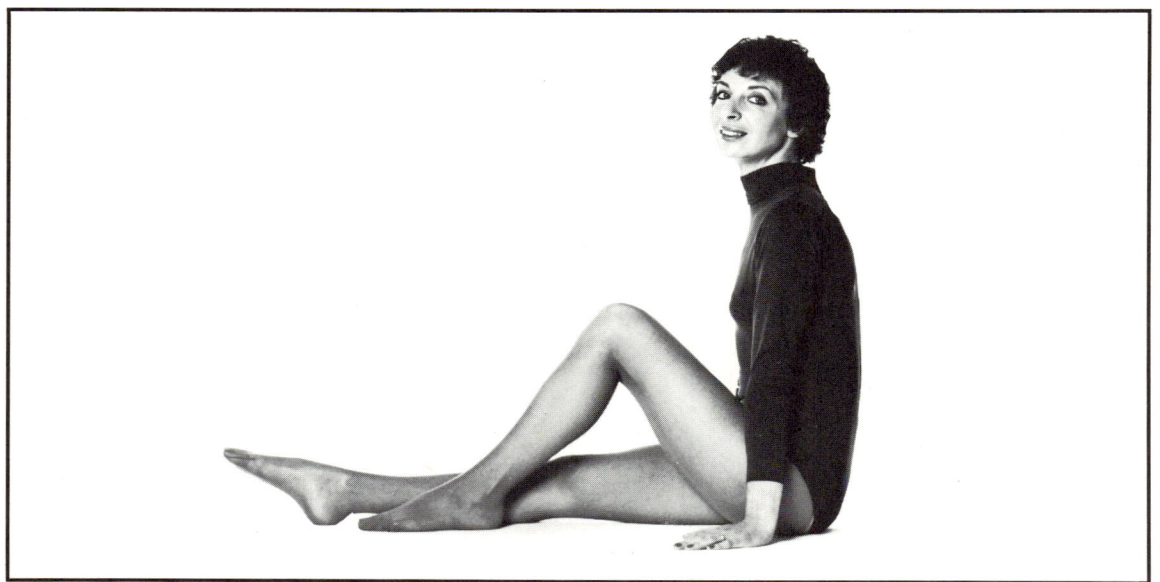

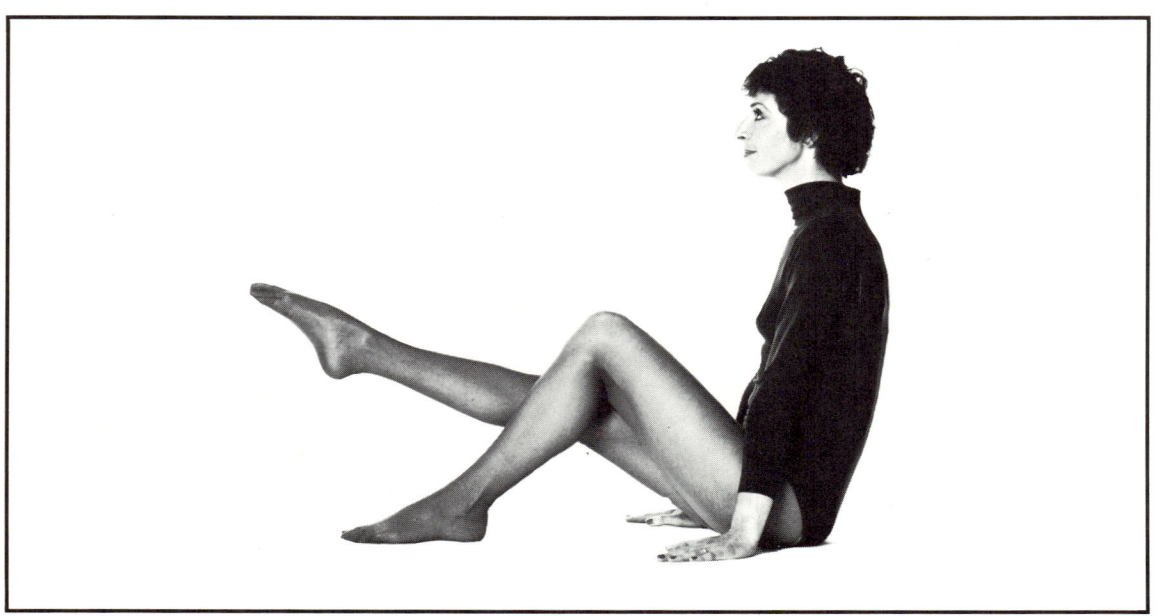

stretched leg as high as you can (probably not very high to begin with, but no matter as just the effort will pull up your stomach muscles and also work your thighs as you raise your leg). Lower your leg to the floor. Raise and lower your stretched leg five times then change over and do the other leg.

2.** This is a much tougher variation. Sit on the floor with both knees bent and feet on the floor. Hands still placed at either side of you on the floor. Stretch both legs up as high as you can. Hold to the count of five. Bend your knees and place your feet back on the floor. Repeat several times.

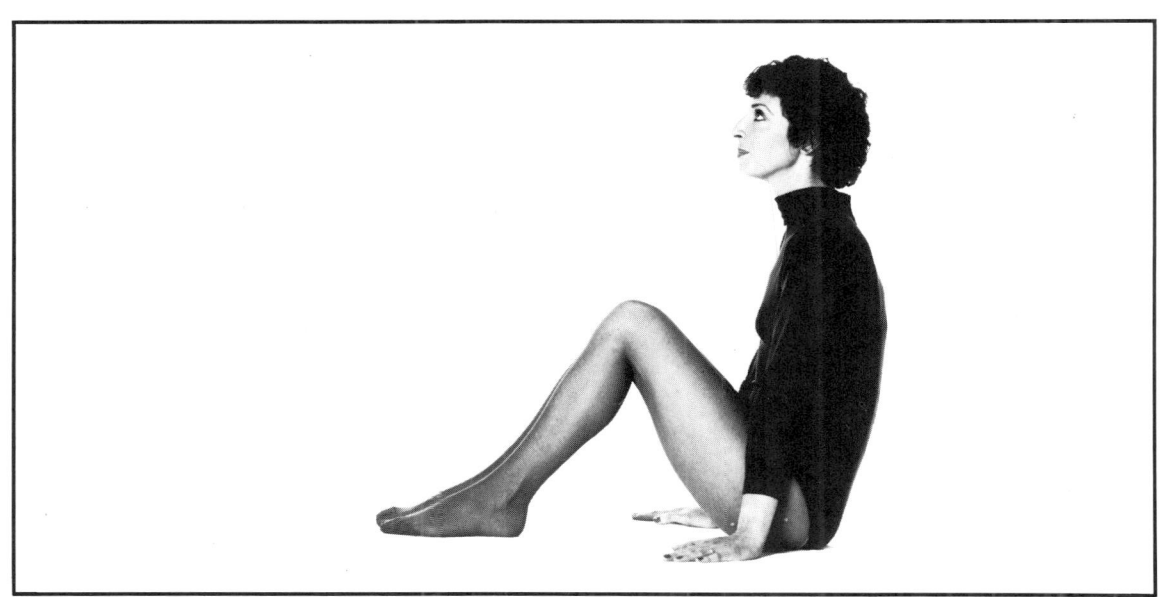

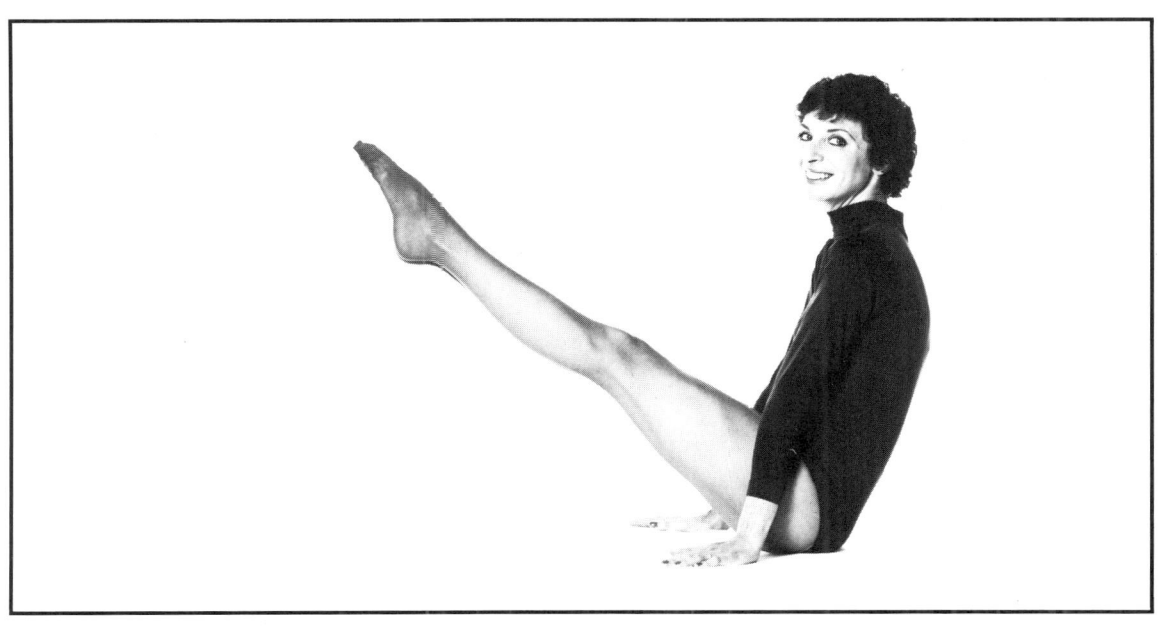

THE STOMACH & THIGHS II

This exercise is particularly good for the lower stomach and the upper thighs.

1.*** Sit with your bottom pushed right against the back of a kitchen chair, and your legs apart. Grip the edge of the front of your chair between your legs.

Lift both legs out in front of you with your feet turned up so that your toes face towards the ceiling.

Keep your legs taut and do not allow them to drop. Pump your feet and legs up towards the ceiling five times. The more of your legs that leave the chair the greater the muscle work you are achieving.

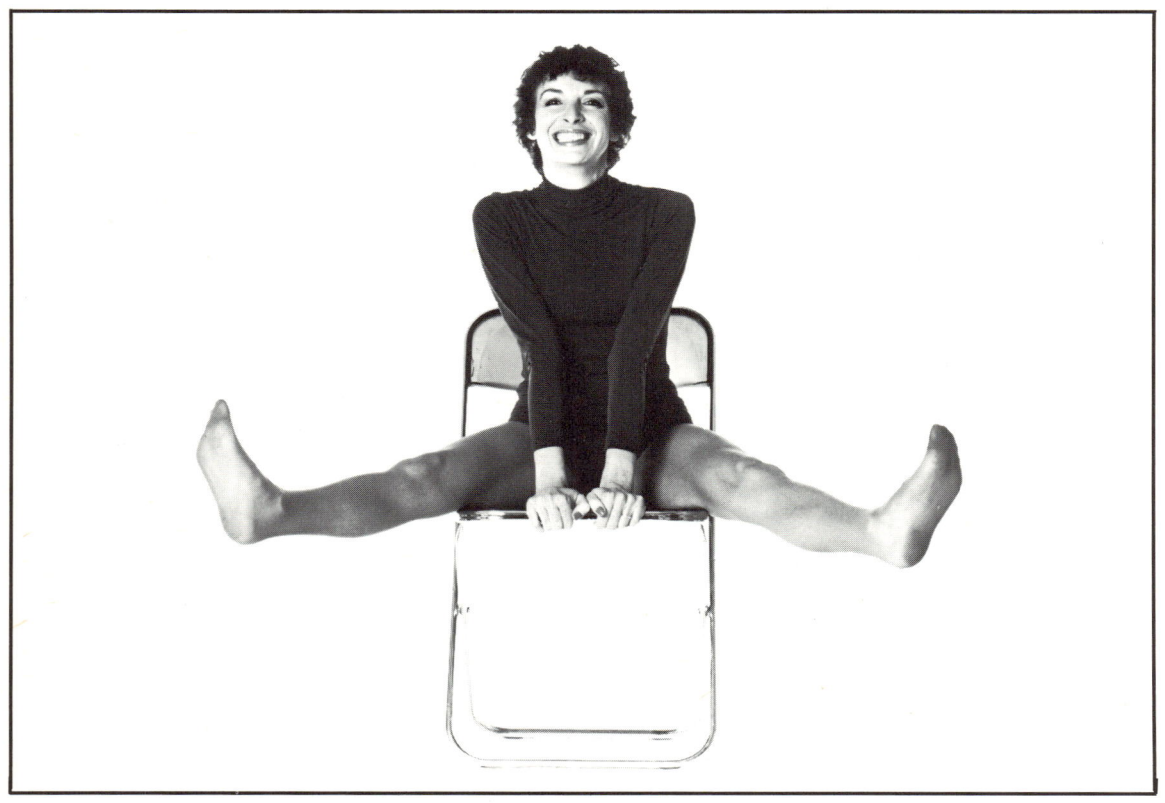

THE STOMACH AND THIGHS

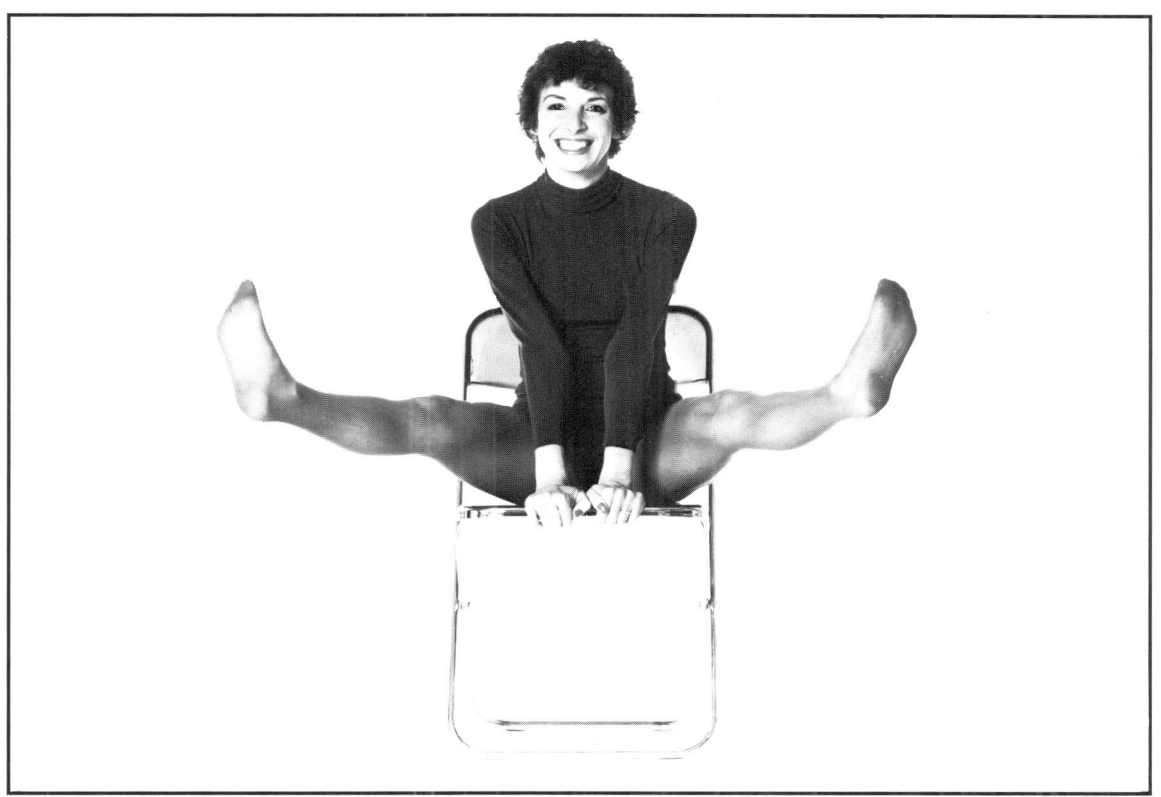

THE STOMACH & THIGHS III

This exercise is good for your stomach and thigh muscles, and the higher you can raise your legs the more your stomach muscles have to work and the sooner you will firm them up. But do make sure you have worked on a few of the other, easier, stomach exercises before attempting this one.

1.**** Sit on the edge of a kitchen chair and lean back with your shoulders against the back of the chair. Grip the edge of the seat behind you with your hands. Bend your knees lifting them up as near to your chest as possible.

Stretch your legs out in front of you keeping your legs together and beautifully stretched right through to your toes. Repeat the bending and stretching of your legs five times if you can.

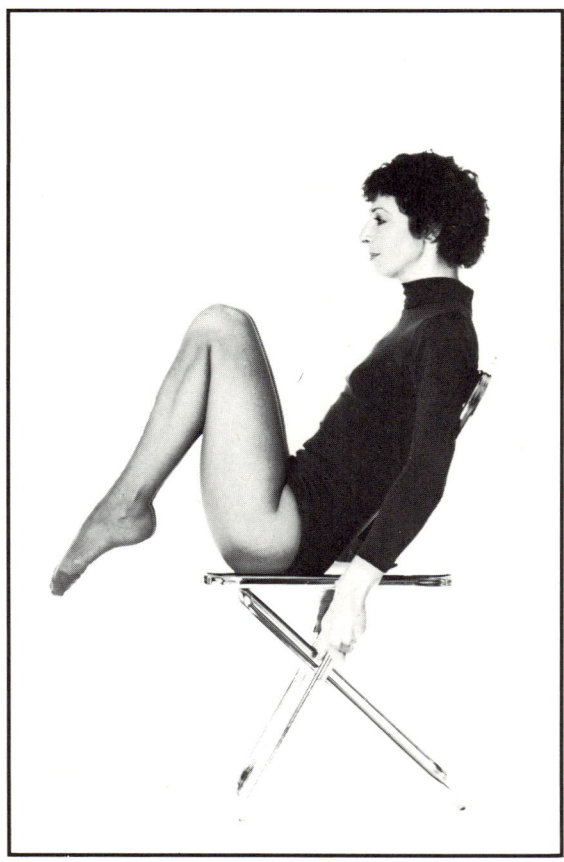

THE STOMACH AND THIGHS 73

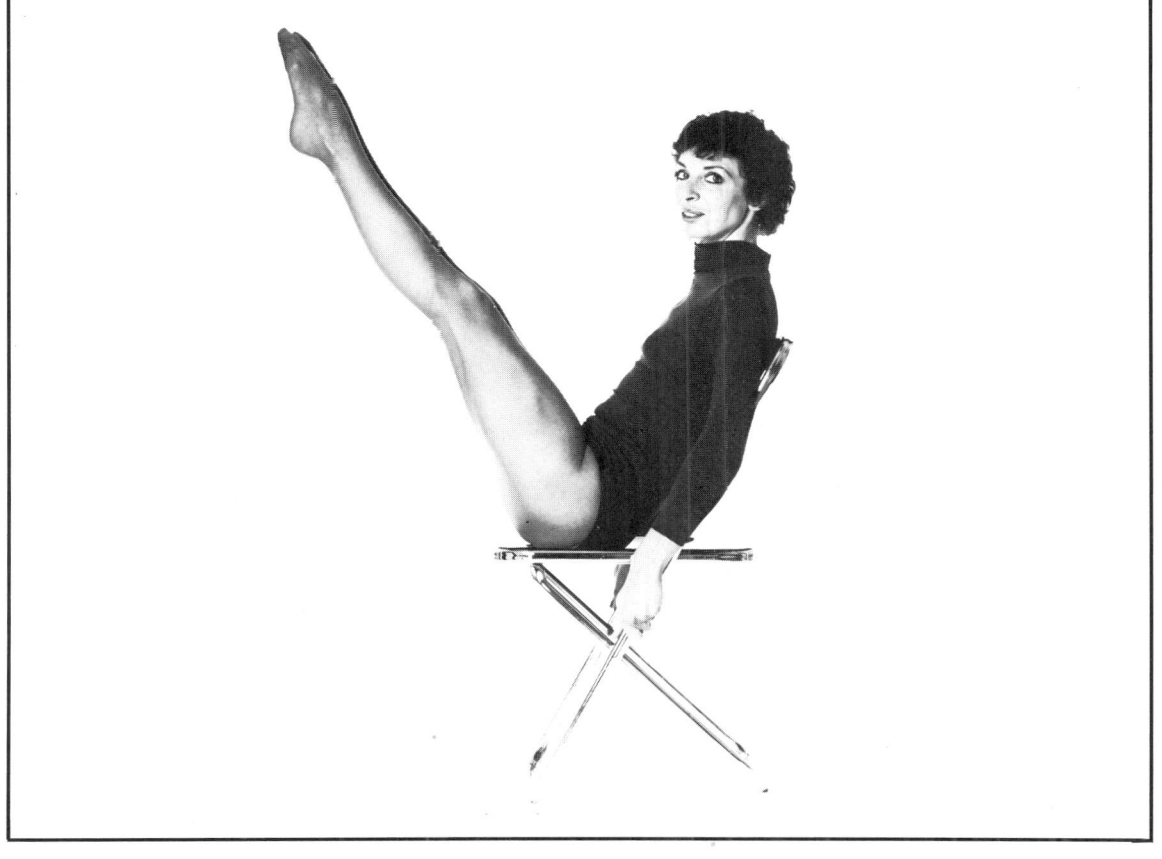

THE STOMACH & THIGHS IV

The Sink Special 1

This way of exercising is excellent and really works the greater part of your body, virtually from top to toe. All you need is a sink for support and heaps of effort. Once you have mastered this particular way of exercising there are many variations, and I'm confident that by using your imagination you could invent some fine new exercises to do yourself and share with your friends. Remember an exercise morning with friends can be lots of fun and far less fattening than a coffee and cakes morning.

1.★ Sit down on the floor with your shoulders comfortably leaning against the sink unit, and your bottom about twelve inches from the unit.

Bring your arms up and over your head and grip the lip of the sink with your hands so that your fingers curl into the sink.

Lift one leg up as high as you can. Hold it. Place it back on the floor and repeat the movement with your other leg. Keep your legs fully stretched right through to a beautifully pointed toe.

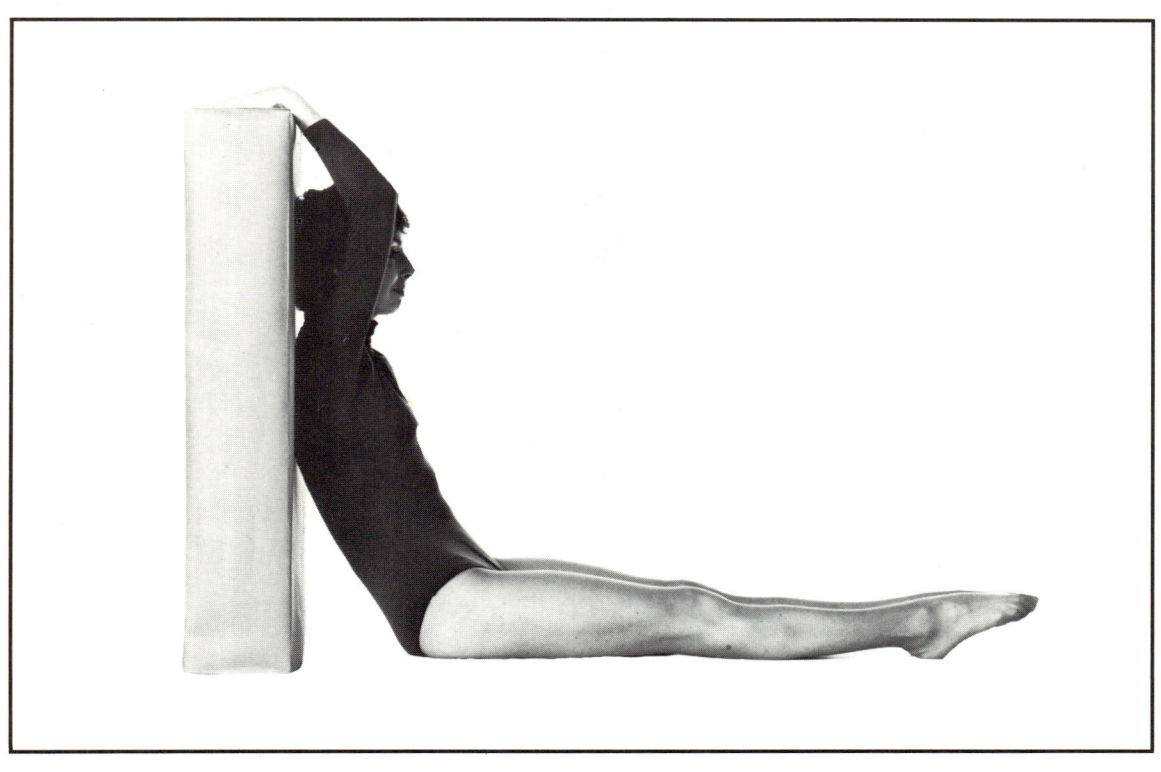

THE STOMACH AND THIGHS

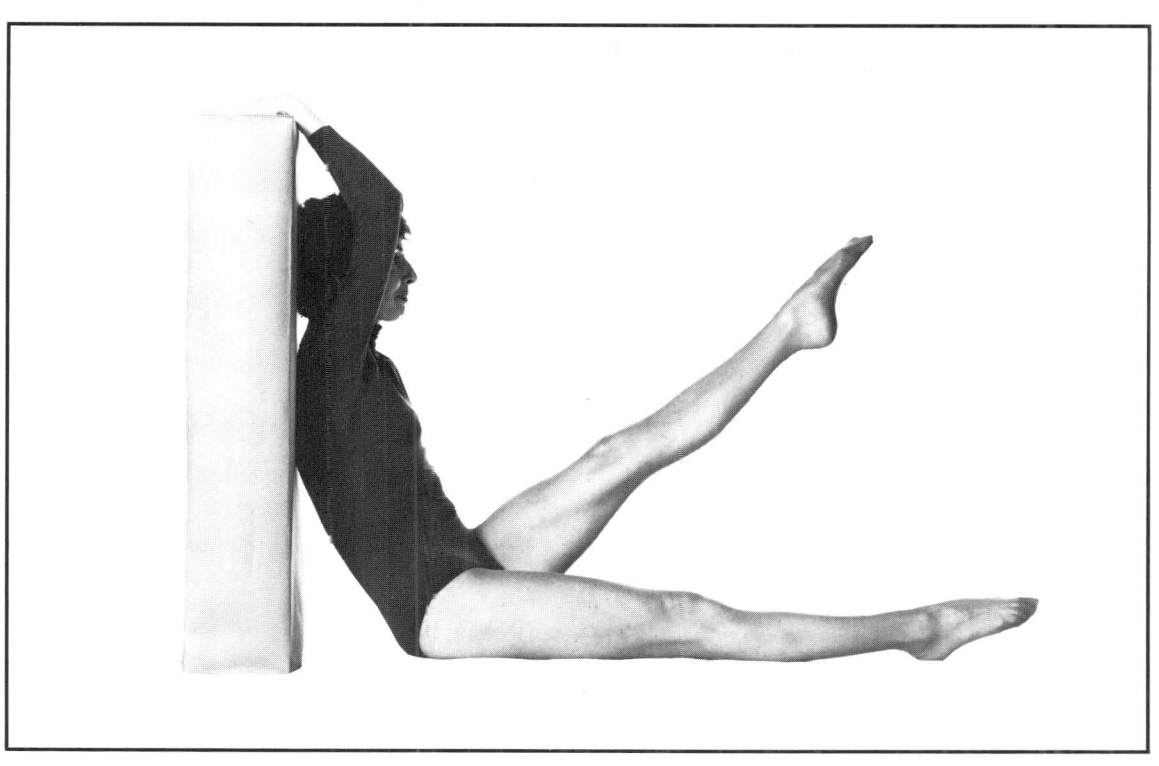

THE STOMACH & THIGHS V

The Sink Special 2

You can make this exercise a little tougher by working with your legs apart.

1.** Sit on the floor against your sink unit as in the preceding exercise. Lift one leg up. Then the other so that they are together. Lower one leg, then the other. Keep legs stretched right through to your toes. Repeat several times.

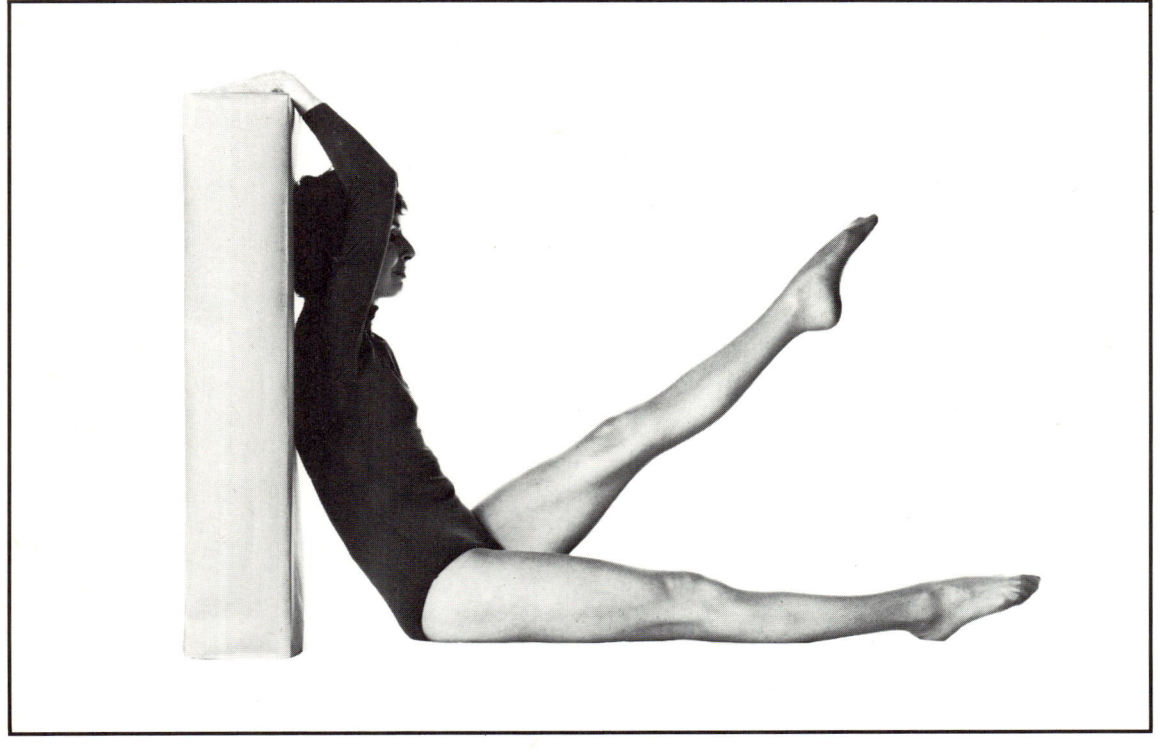

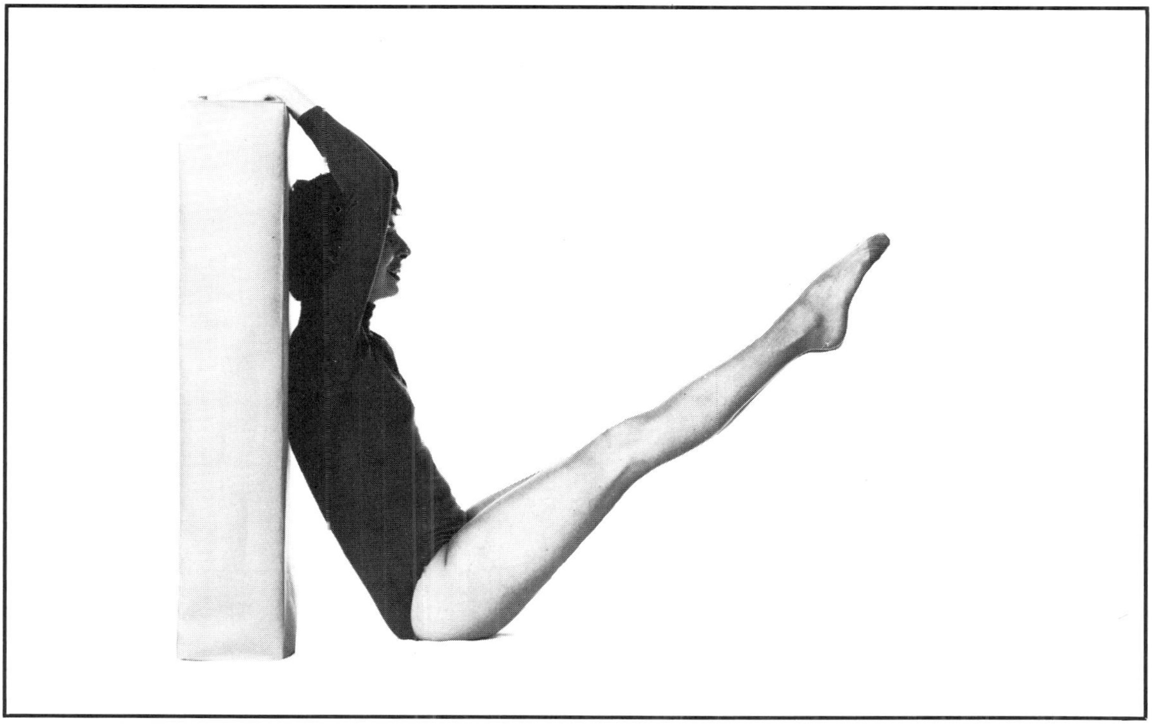

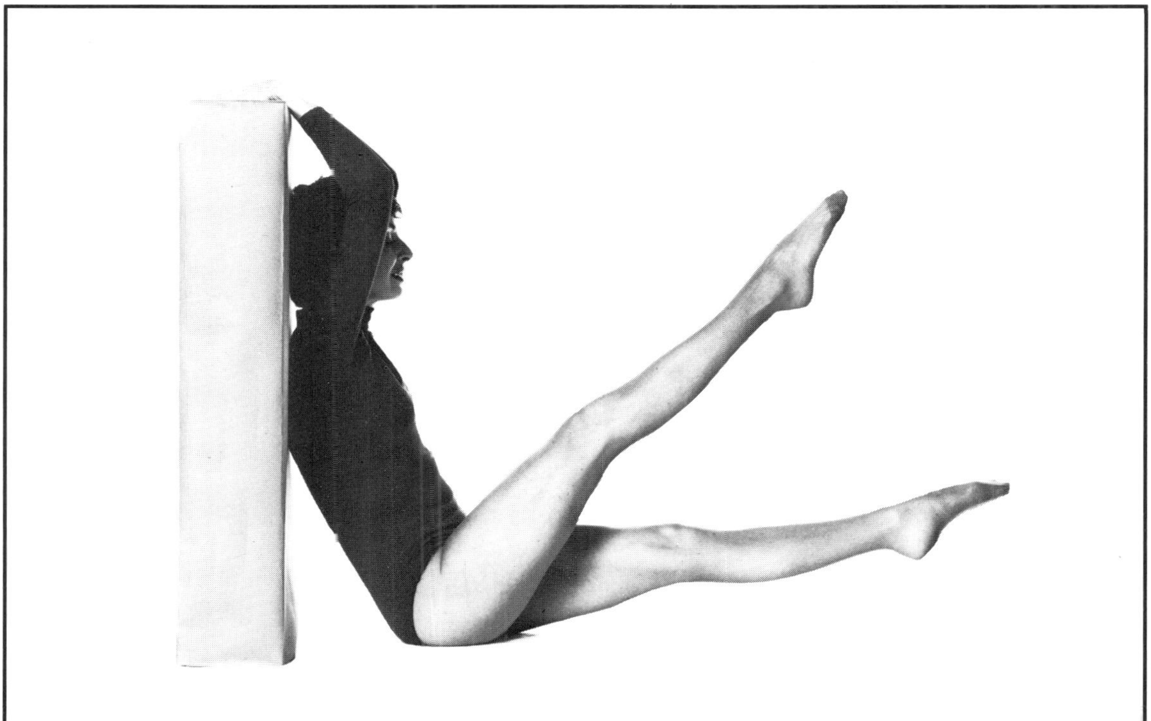

THE STOMACH AND THIGHS

THE STOMACH & THIGHS VI

The Sink Special 3

This is a really marvellous exercise done slowly or fast, and it's number one for firming you up from top to toe.

1.*** Sit on the floor against your sink unit as in *Sink Special 1*.

Grip the sink firmly with your hands. Keeping your legs together raised off the floor, begin to walk with your legs. Make nice big strides. Keep your legs stretched and toes pointed. If your knees bend, you're cheating!

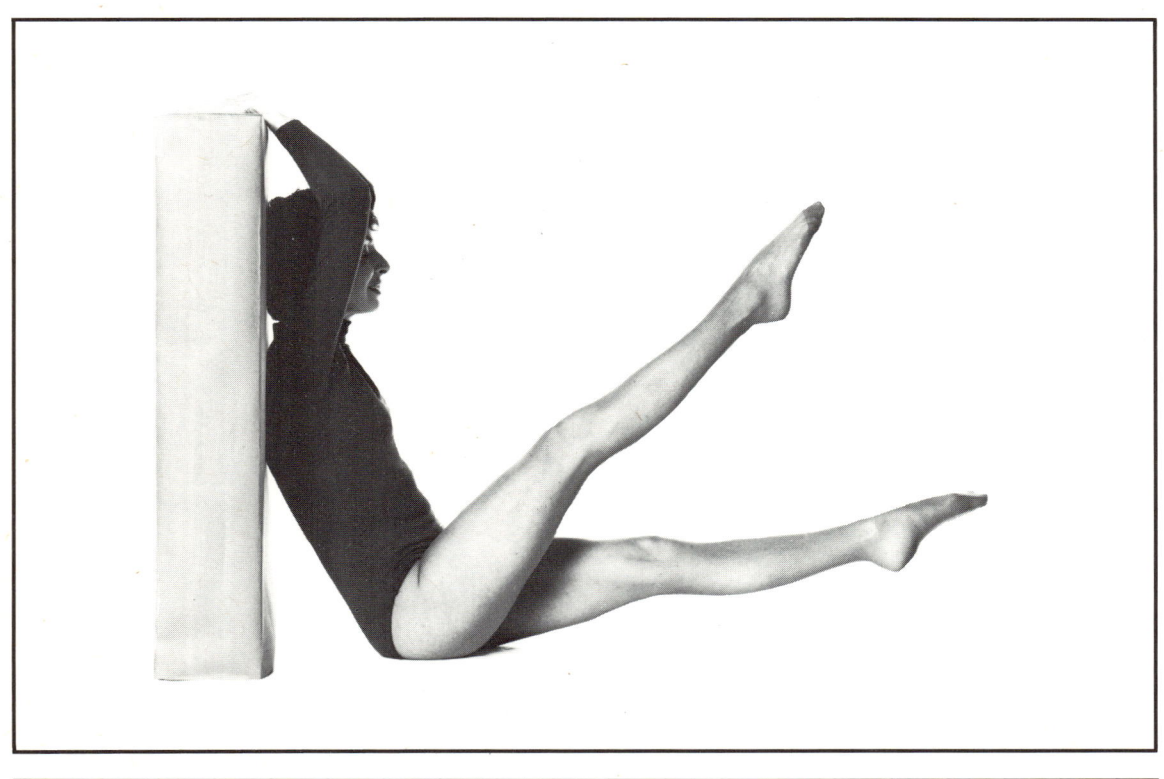

The Sink Special 4

If you can ultimately achieve ten of these movements, full marks, because your stomach and thigh muscles will most certainly be strong and firm.

1.**** Sit down against your sink unit as in the preceding exercises, with your legs apart and stretched right out. Grip the sink firmly with your hands. Raise your legs as high as possible and watch your knees to check that they don't bend.

Open and close your legs. Start with three times and work up until you can manage ten comfortably.

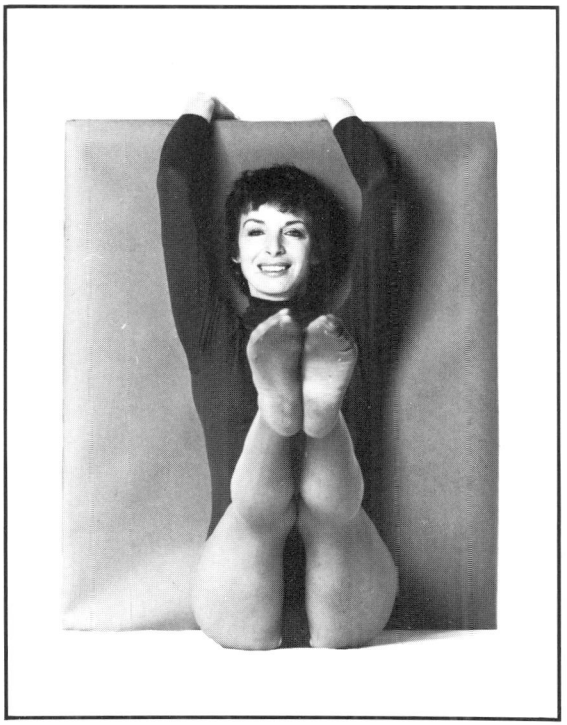

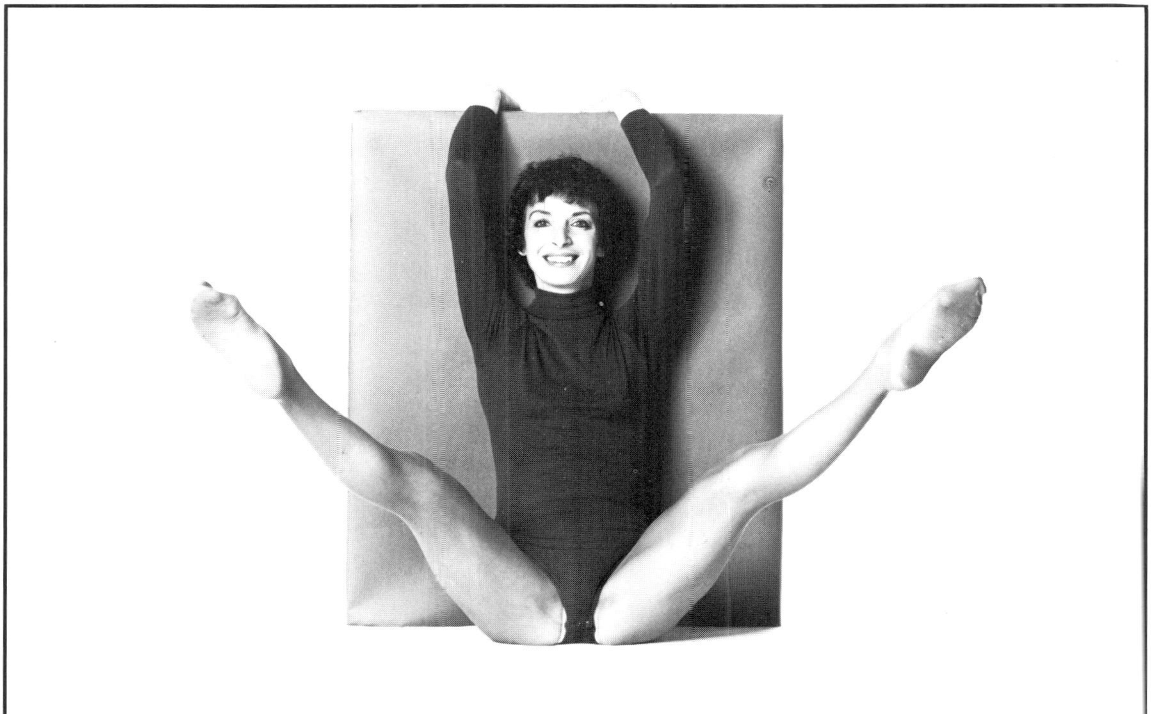

THE STOMACH & THIGHS VII

The Sink Special 5

When you can do this exercise ten times or more, you will have conquered one of the toughest exercises and can be duly proud.

1.***** Sit down against your sink unit as in the preceding exercises, with your legs stretched right out but together.

Grip the sink with your hands. Raise your legs as high as you can and then lower them to within an inch of the floor. Do not allow your feet to touch the floor. Raise them again as high as possible. To begin with, do this exercise twice only. You can aim for more and achieve more as you become stronger.

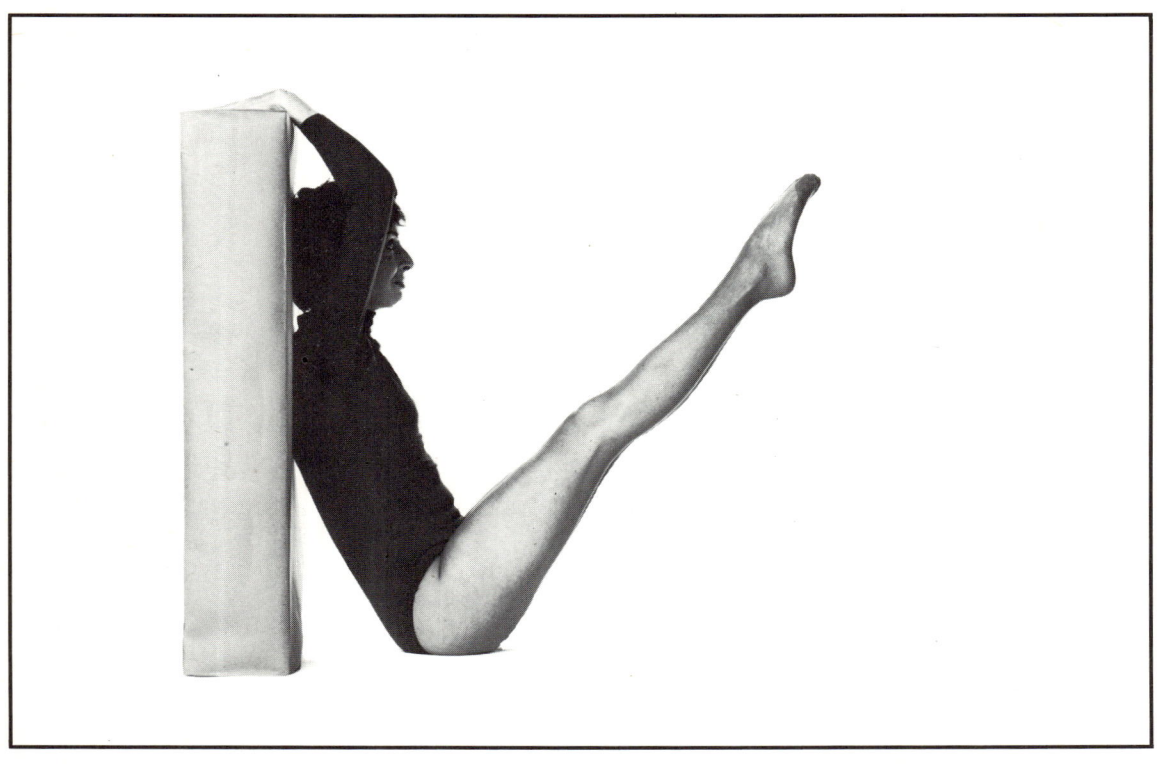

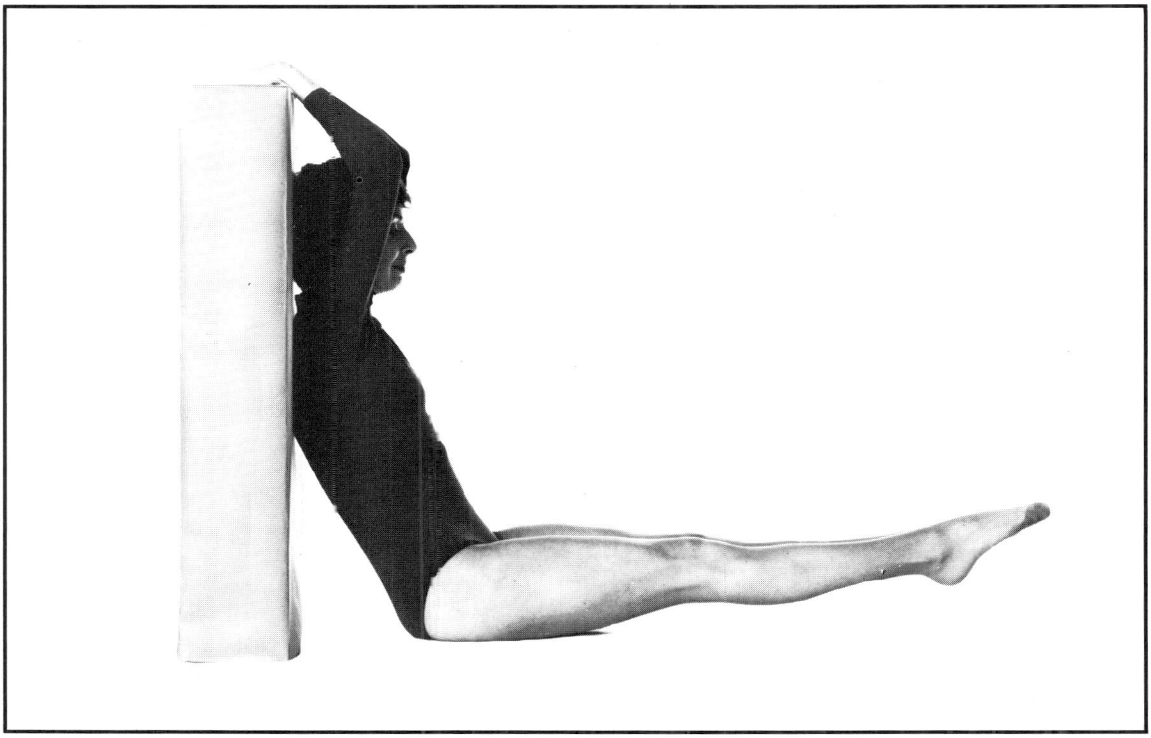

THE STOMACH AND THIGHS

THE THIGHS

If you've followed any of the exercises in the preceding section for the Stomach and Thighs, your thighs should be progressing, and the muscles firming up.

There are two sets of muscles in the thighs, which, if unused, can contribute to unsightly flab and fat. The outside thighs can develop 'handles', and the inner thighs, like the upper arms, can start to look loose and bobbly. Both sets of muscles need vigorous and constant attention in the form of exercises, so that the thighs can look trim and healthy.

THE THIGHS I

This exercise is particularly good for the upper inside of the thighs which can become extremely flabby, in much the same way as the upper arm. If you are overweight, this can even cause discomfort.

1.★ Place a kitchen chair in the centre of the room. Lie on your back close enough to the chair so that you can place the instep of your feet around the legs of the chair six inches from the floor. Now squeeze the legs of the chair as hard as

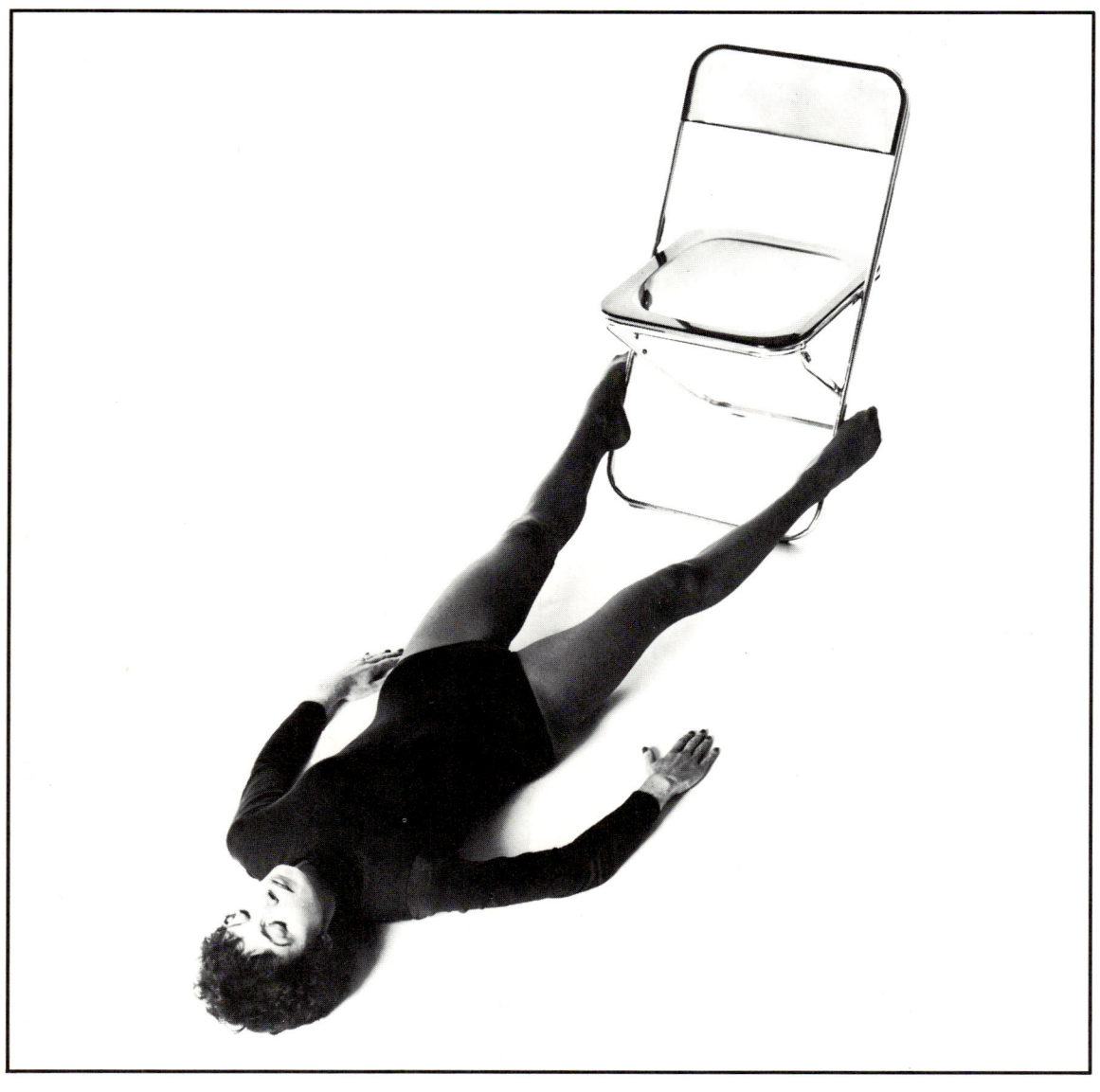

you can for the count of ten. (Of course, using the legs of your husband or wife or a good friend is much more comfortable on your feet!) Raising your head and shoulders off the floor is good for your stomach as well.

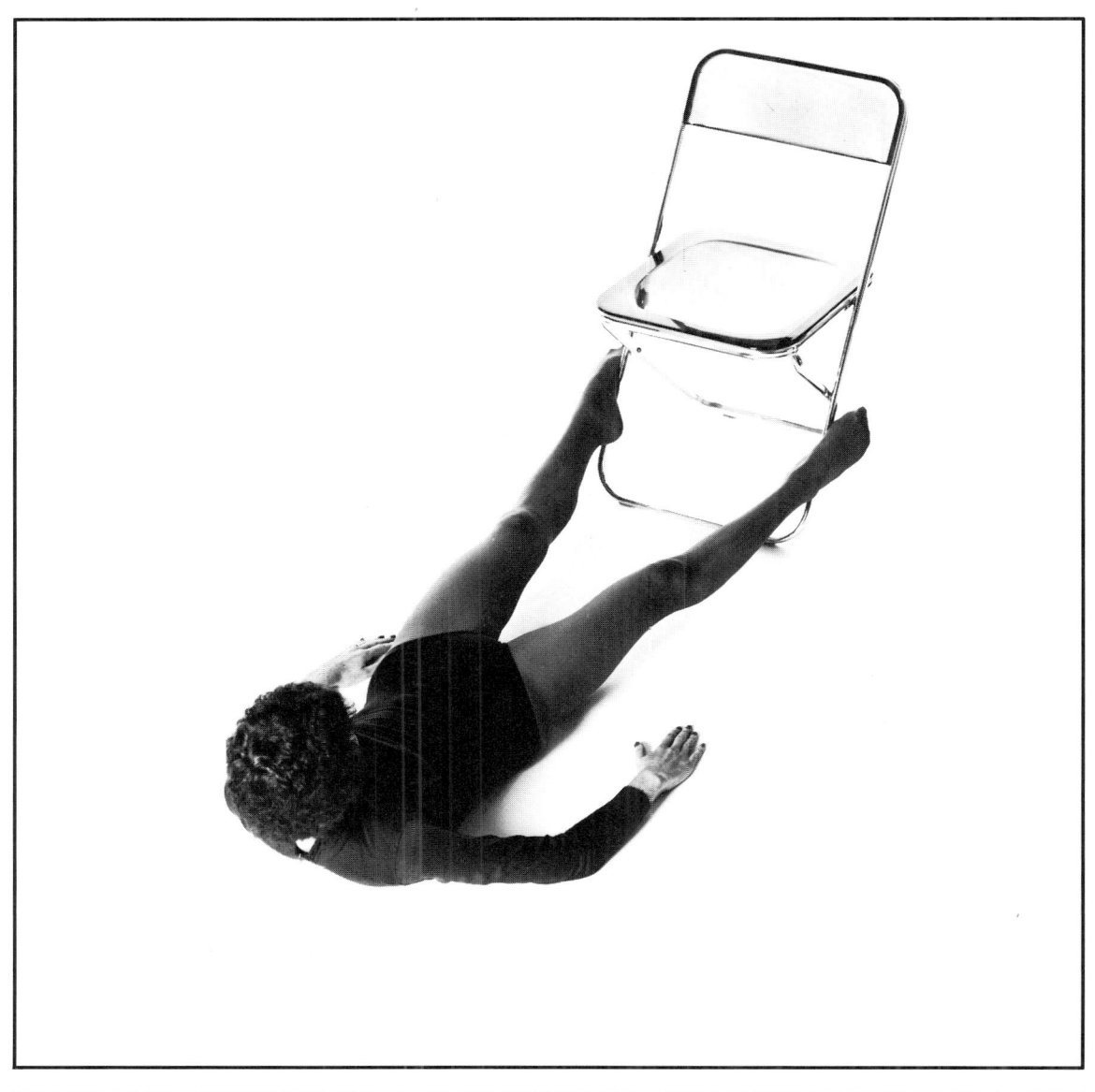

THE THIGHS II

If you have any sort of back complaint, don't do this exercise, or at least consult your doctor first. For a normal healthy body it's excellent, though, and will give your spine a lovely stretch while also stretching and firming the inner thigh muscles.

1.* Sit on the floor with your legs well apart and your feet turned up so that your toes are pointing towards the ceiling.

Lean forward with your arms stretched in front of you as though trying to grasp something just out of your reach. Don't curve your back, but lean over from your hip joint keeping your back as straight as possible.

Pump forward getting lower and lower. Keep your knees locked and straight, which is very good for the firming up of the inner thigh, and you should be able to feel the muscles here working as you pump forward.

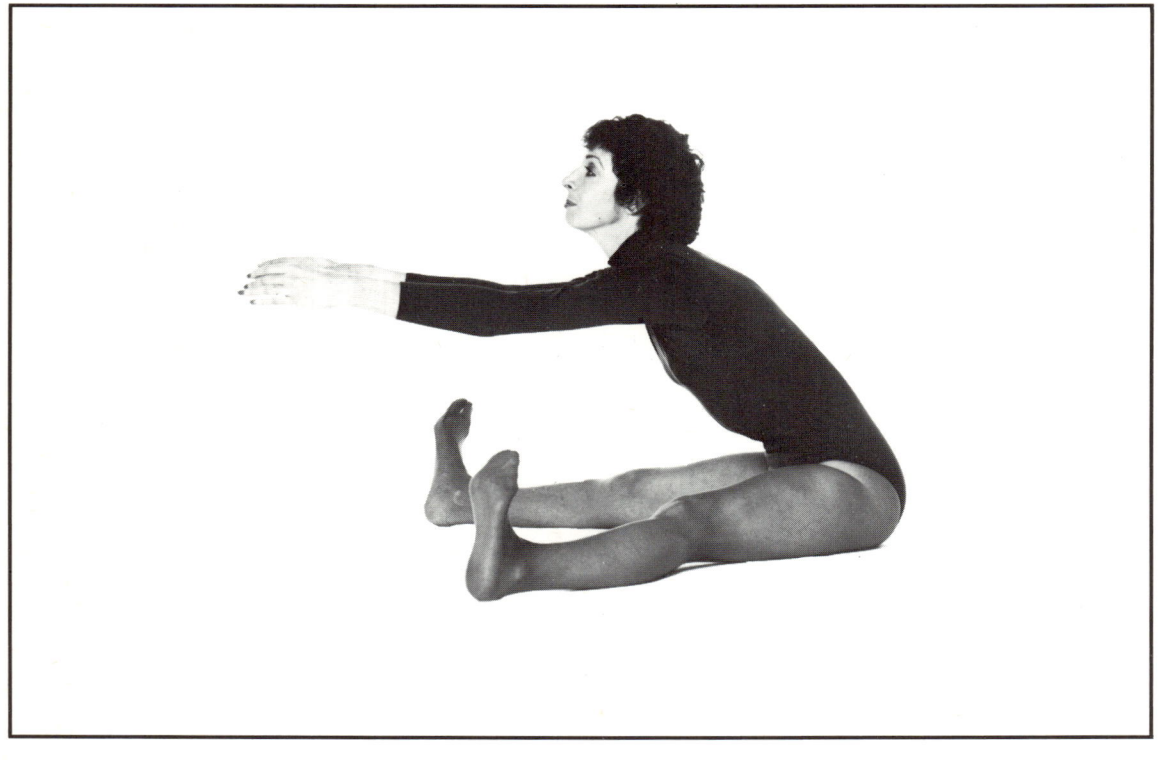

THE THIGHS 87

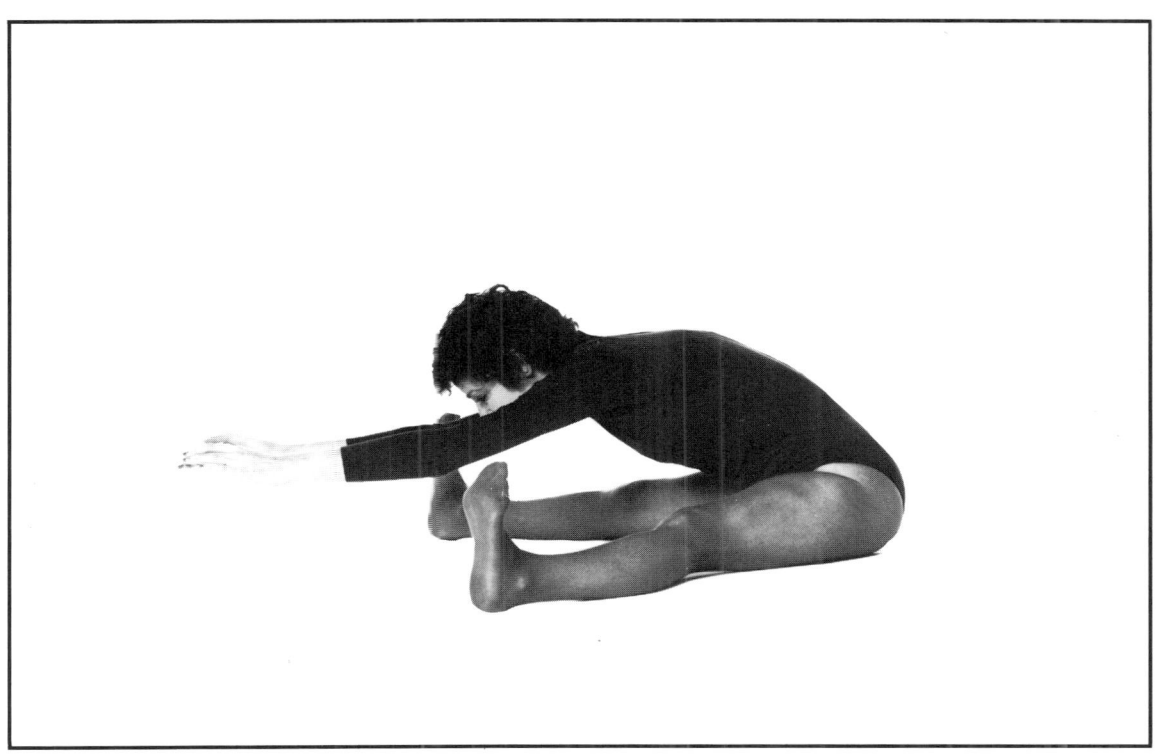

THE THIGHS III

This exercise firms up both sets of muscles in the outstretched leg.

1.★ Stand side-ways to your sink which will take the strain while you use it for support.

Grip sink firmly with one hand and lift your outside leg out to the side as high as you can. Keep your leg beautifully stretched and point your toe.

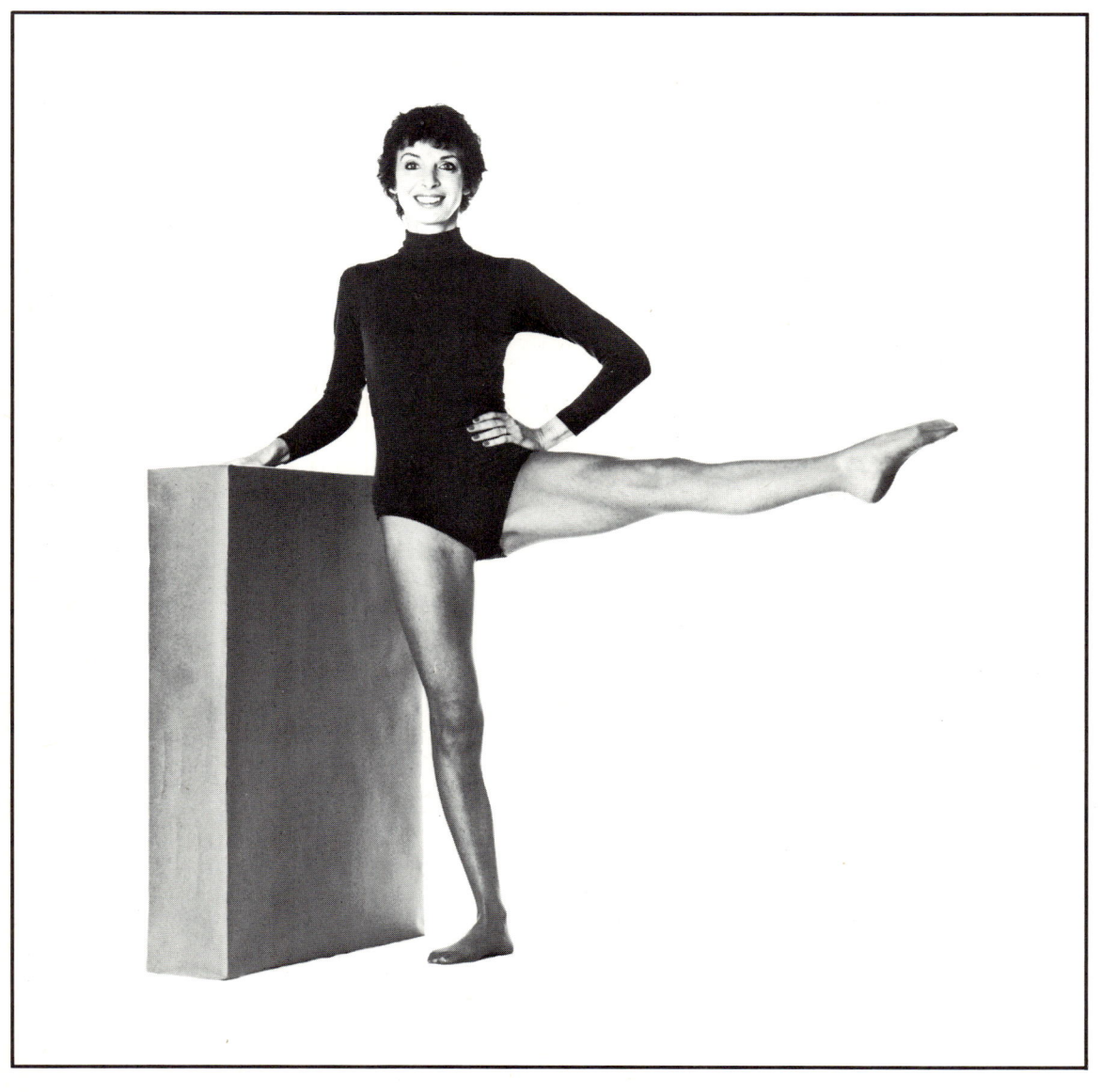

Bend and stretch your outside leg five times (more once you become stronger). Then turn round and do the other leg.

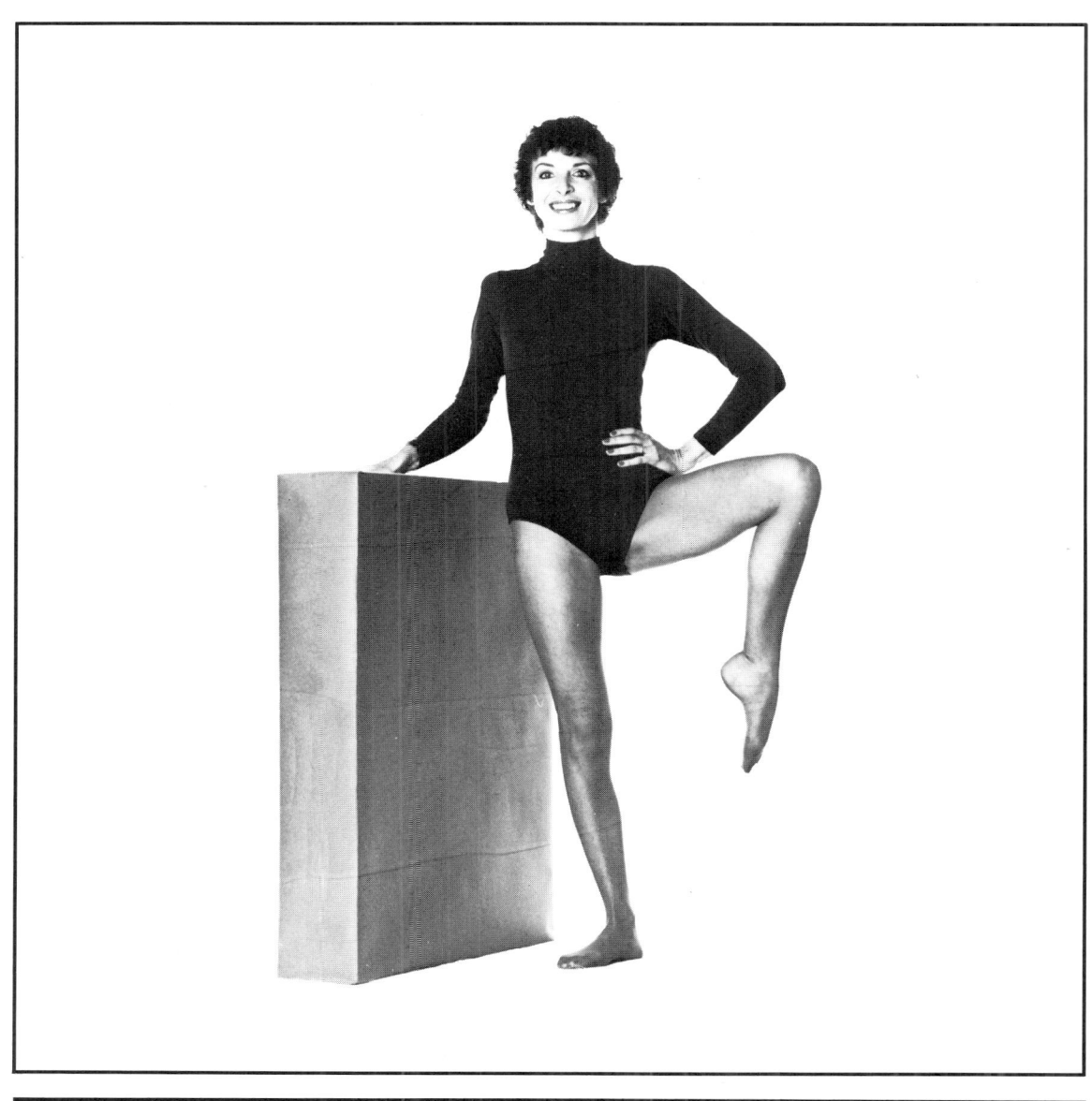

THE THIGHS IV

This exercise works on the same muscles as the previous one, but a little more strenuously!

1.** Stand side-ways to your sink and grip it firmly with one hand for support. Lift the outside leg out to your side keeping your leg very straight, and this time turn your foot so that your toe is pointing to the ceiling.

Pump your leg up ten times as though you were trying to touch the ceiling with your toe. Be sure to keep the knees of

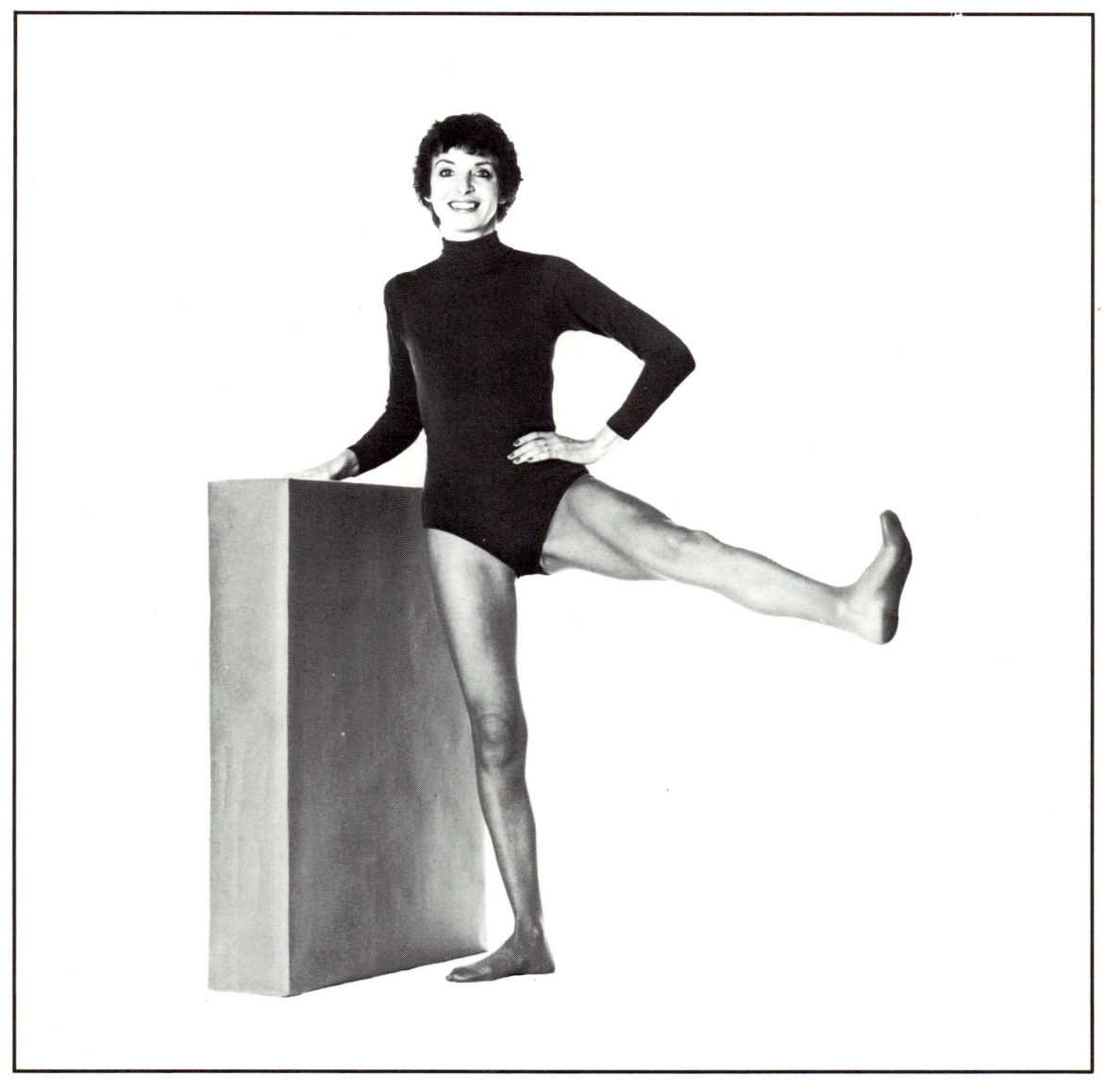

both your legs locked, and don't allow the leg you are pumping to drop. The emphasis is on the UP.

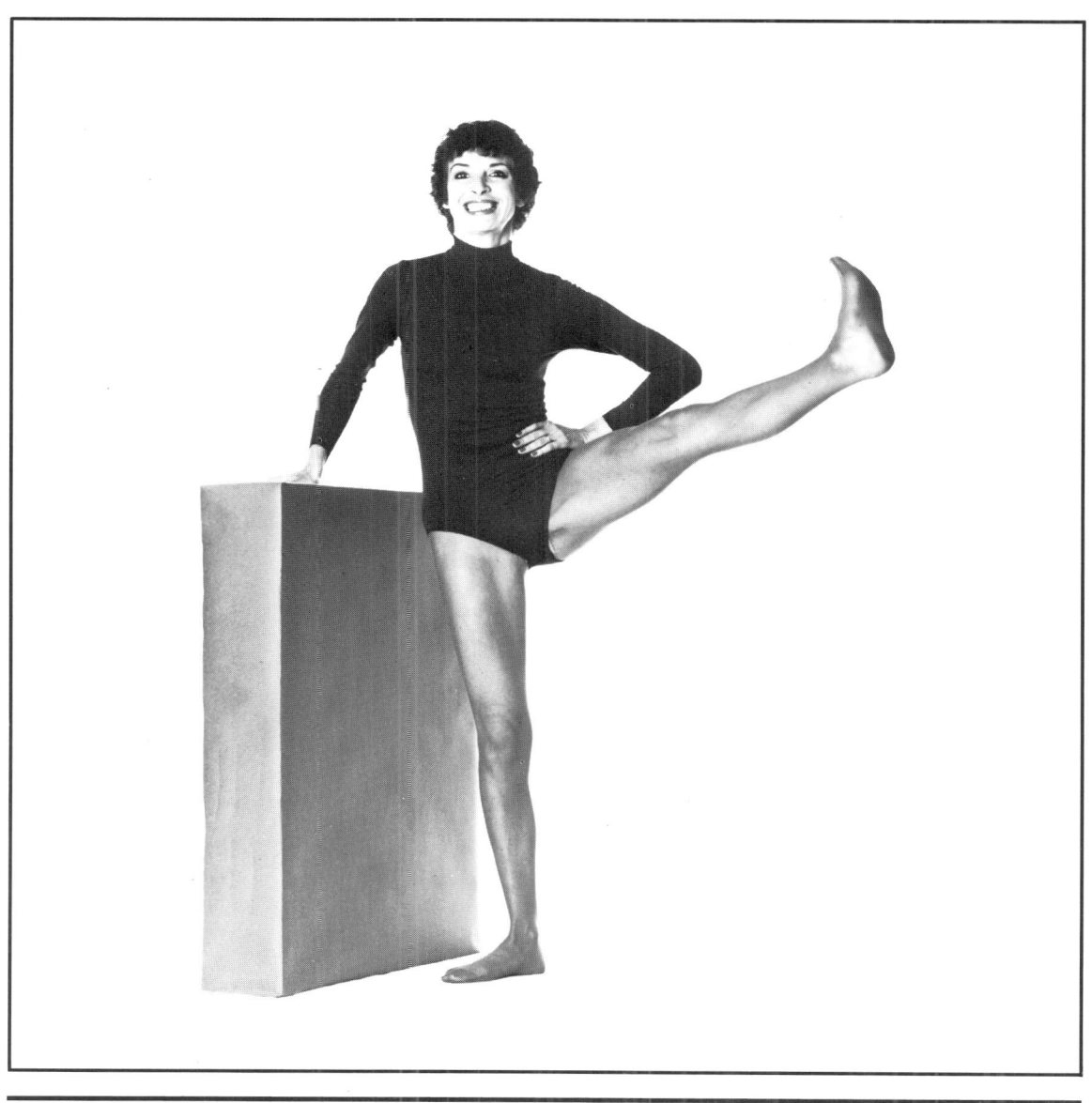

THE THIGHS V

This exercise is full of strain at first, but if you persevere, and work up towards ten sit-ups, you will never have to worry about flabby thighs again.

1.**** Stand side-ways to your kitchen sink and grip with one hand. Feet together. Rise up onto the balls of your feet.

Go right down allowing your knees to part as you go down until your bottom touches your heels. Remember to stay on the balls of your feet and keep your back straight throughout this exercise.

Rise up to the height of a chair seat. Hold this position for the count of five.

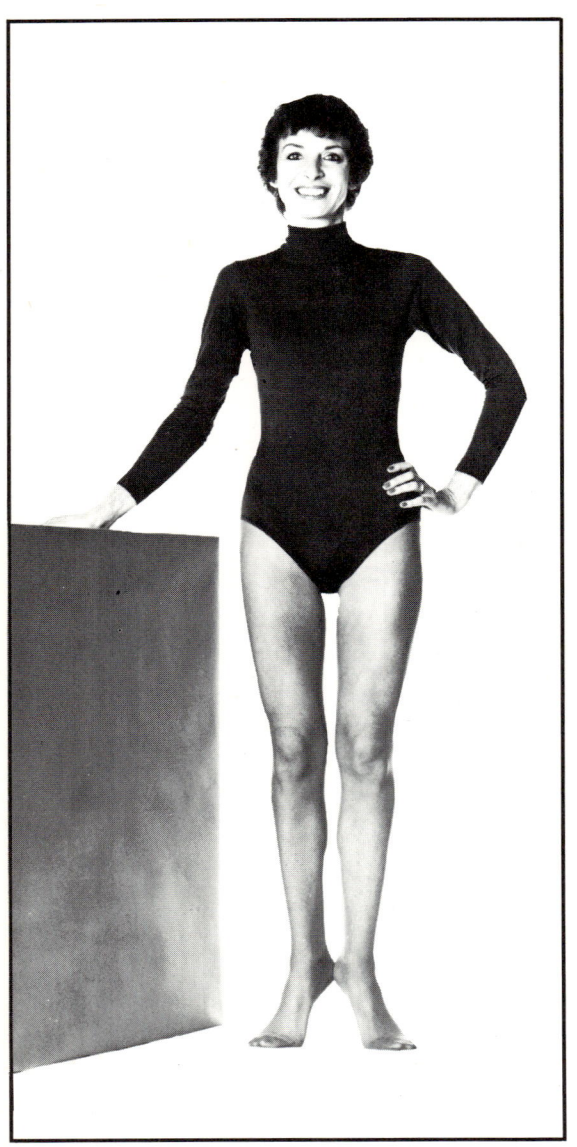

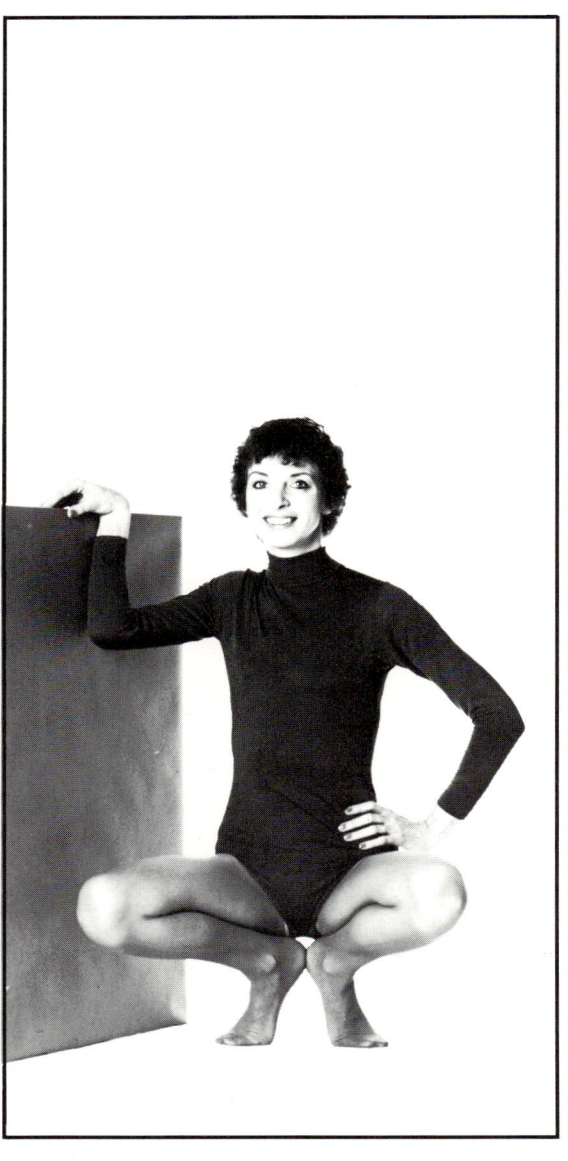

Down again to touch your heels with your bottom. As soon as your heels touch your bottom you rise to the chair height and count five again. Start by doing this routine twice.

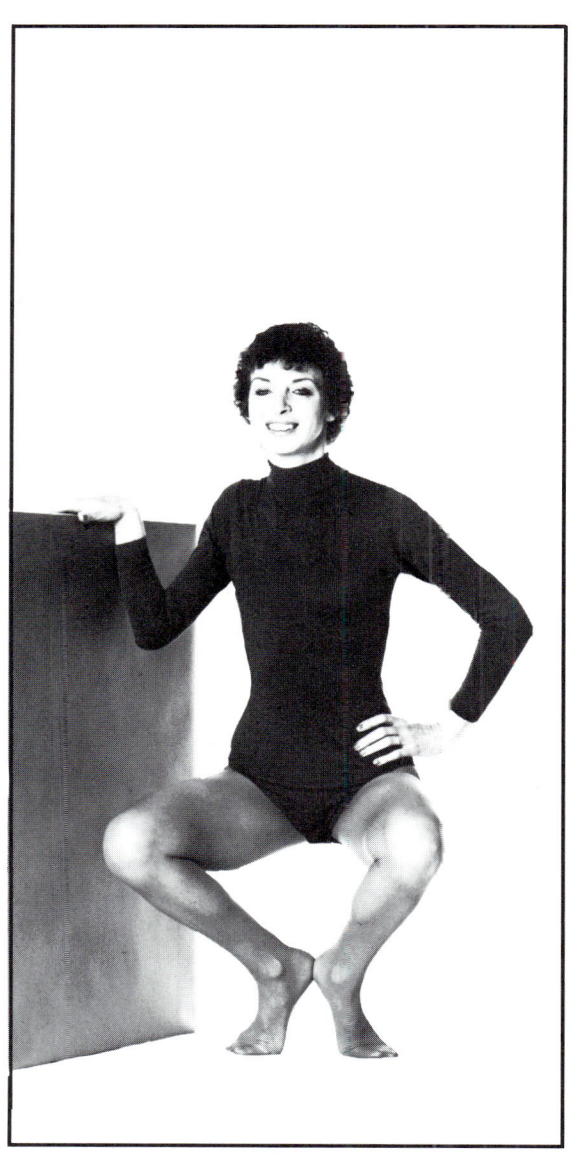

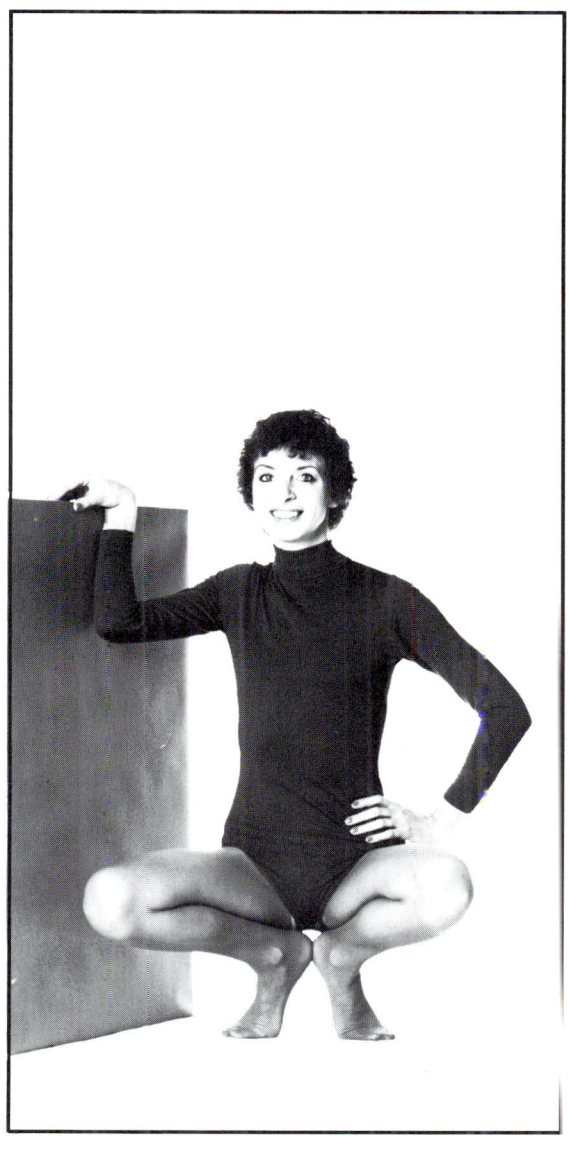

THE BOTTOM

A lot of people I know despair about their bottoms: they're too big, too flabby, too saggy, too low. The bottom does tend to accumulate fat, and it's a fat that just seems to like to stay there. It also spreads, which isn't really surprising as we're always sitting on it. If, like the stomach, we always pulled in the muscles when walking or sitting, the shape and tone of the buttocks would be vastly improved. Watching your weight will, of course, help control the size of your bottom, but plenty of exercise is the best remedy.

THE BOTTOM I

This is a nice simple exercise which will do a lot for your hanging bottom. Within a few months your clothes should feel looser around this area as your muscles firm up. You can't obviously expect to see results overnight, as this depends on the effort, regularity and frequency of your exercises. Do this exercise gently, not vigorously or jerkily.

1.* Lie face down on the floor. Place a small flattish cushion under your pelvis. Fold your arms in front of you so that you can comfortably rest your head on your arms. Bend your knees so that your feet are pointing up to the ceiling.

Lift both your knees off the floor and push your knees up in small pumping movements. Try not to let your knees touch the floor during this exercise. Only do five pumps at a time, then relax.

2. Finish off with the Back Relaxer Exercise, page 46.

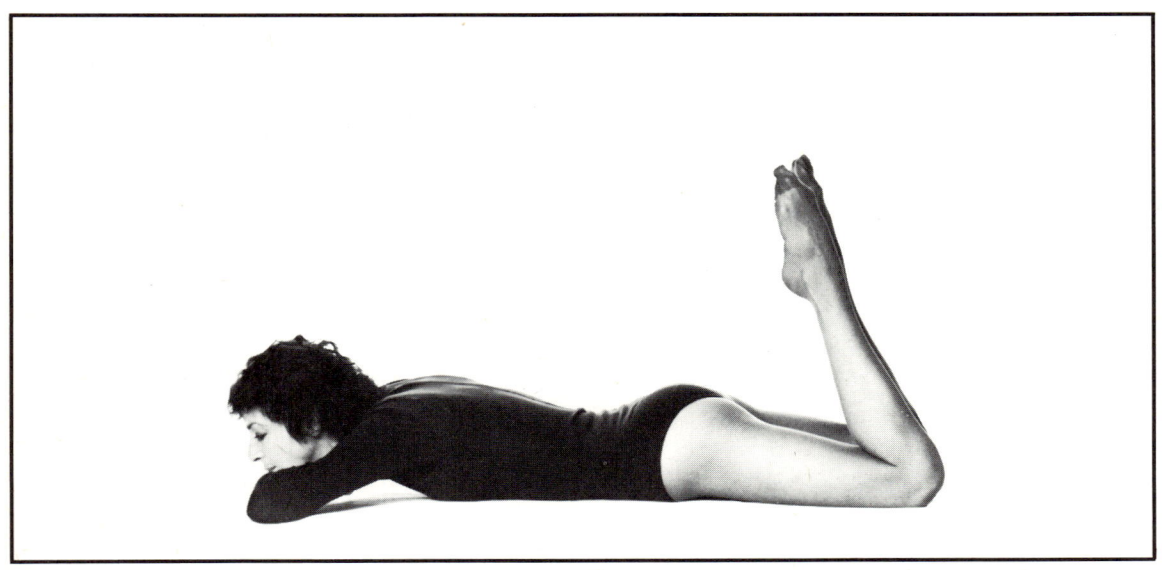

THE BOTTOM 97

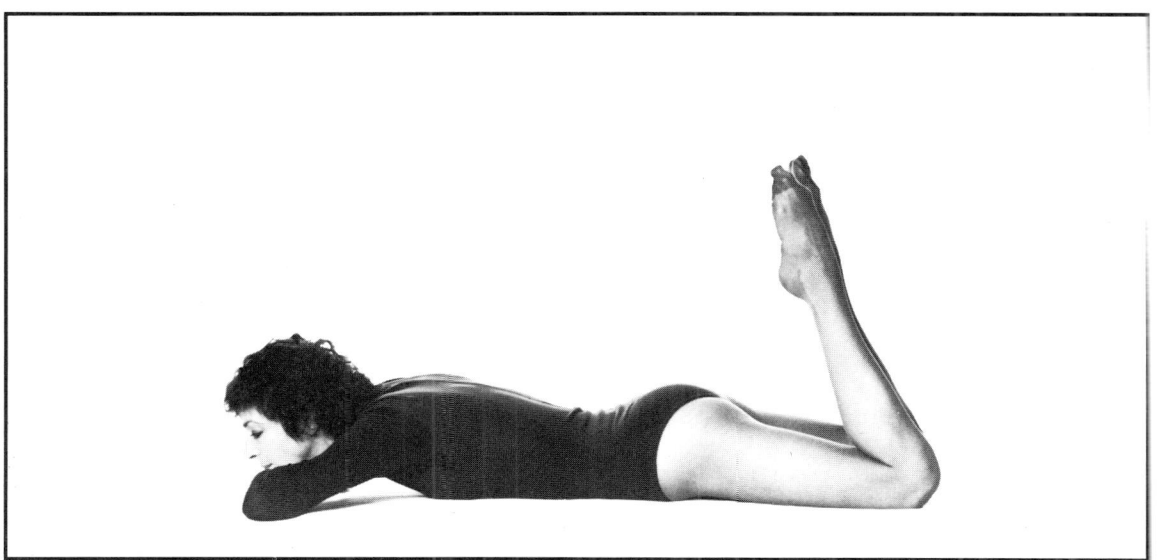

THE BOTTOM II

This exercise is simple and is very good for your buttock and leg muscles.

1.* Stand facing a sturdy surface that you can grip firmly with your hands to give a steady support. The kitchen sink or window-sill would be most suitable provided that there is enough room to stretch your leg out. (The back of a sofa might work as a support.) Move one leg a pace behind, stretching it and pointing your toes. Lift up the outstretched leg keeping your hip pressed against your holding surface. Check that your knees are in the locked position. Hold your leg up for the count of five then replace foot on floor. Repeat several times before changing leg.

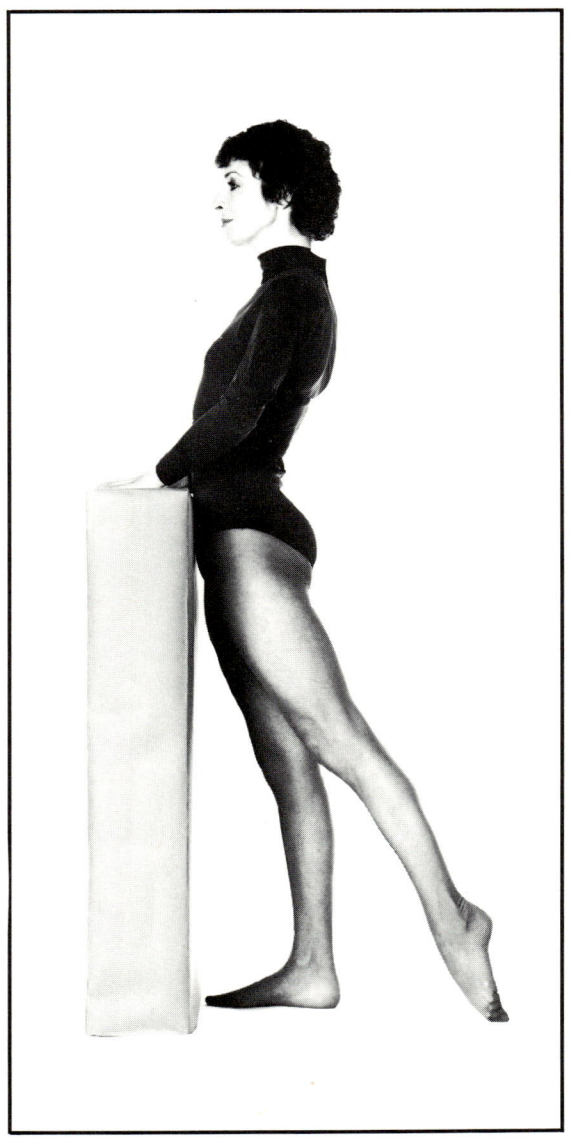

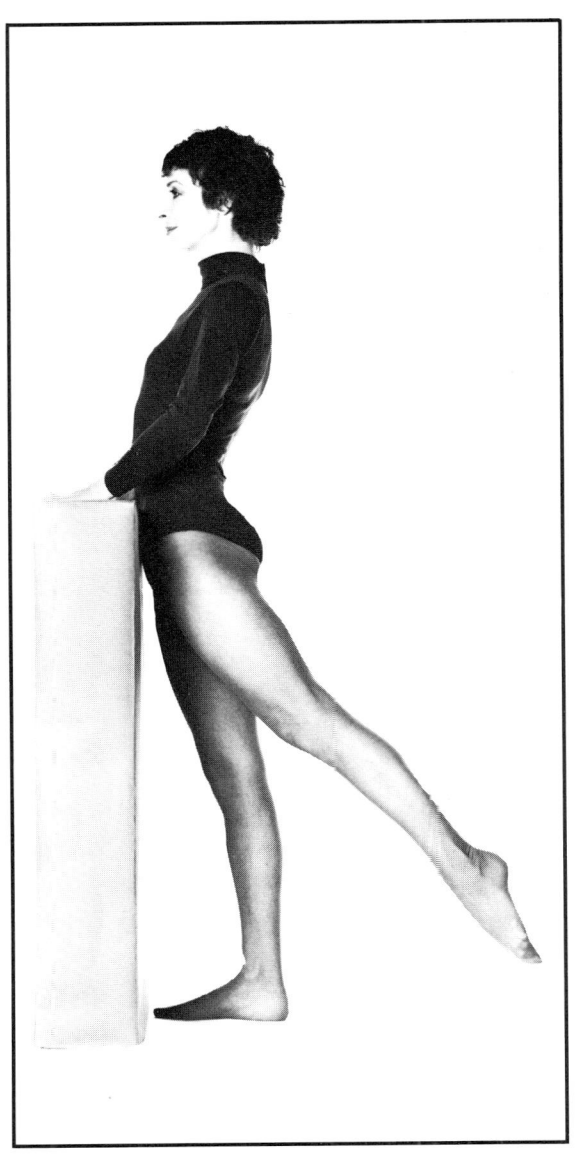

Because you are keeping your hips pressed against your holding surface you will find that you cannot raise your leg very high behind you. This is quite correct and makes the muscles work harder as you try.

THE BOTTOM III

We can become very flabby on the outside of our thighs and hips, and if overweight these parts are prone to accumulate pockets of fat. It's difficult to lose unwanted weight here, but eating wisely and exercising can help trim down unsightly bulges.

1.** Stand as in the previous exercise, facing and holding your supporting surface, but with one leg out to the side. Keep your hip rolled in towards the surface.

Stretch your leg as beautifully as you can and raise it as high as possible. Pump your leg up ten times.

Repeat with your other leg. The more you keep your hip turned in during this exercise the more your hip and thigh will benefit.

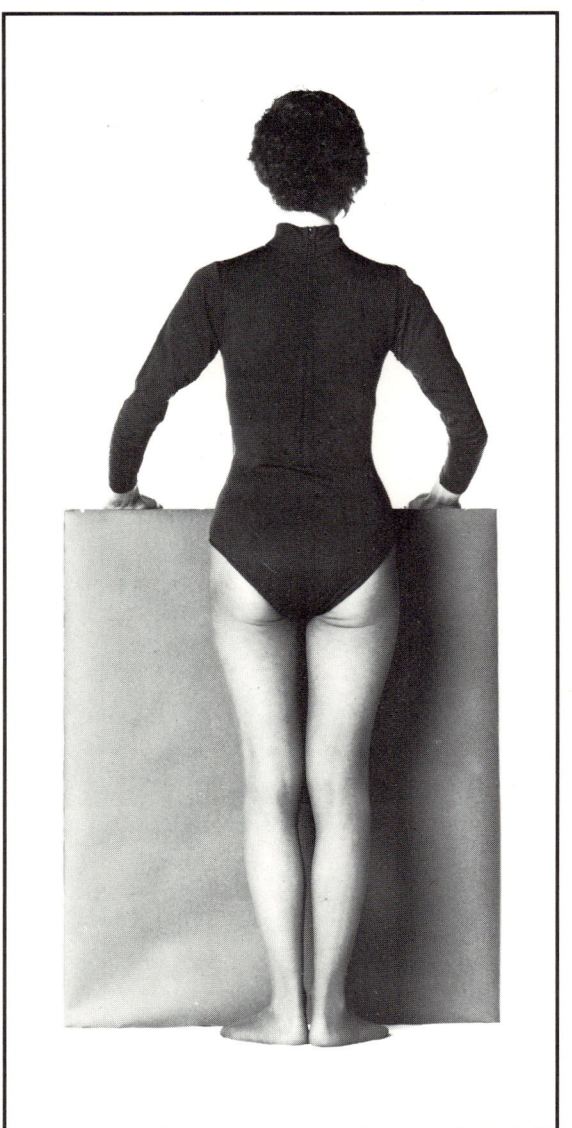

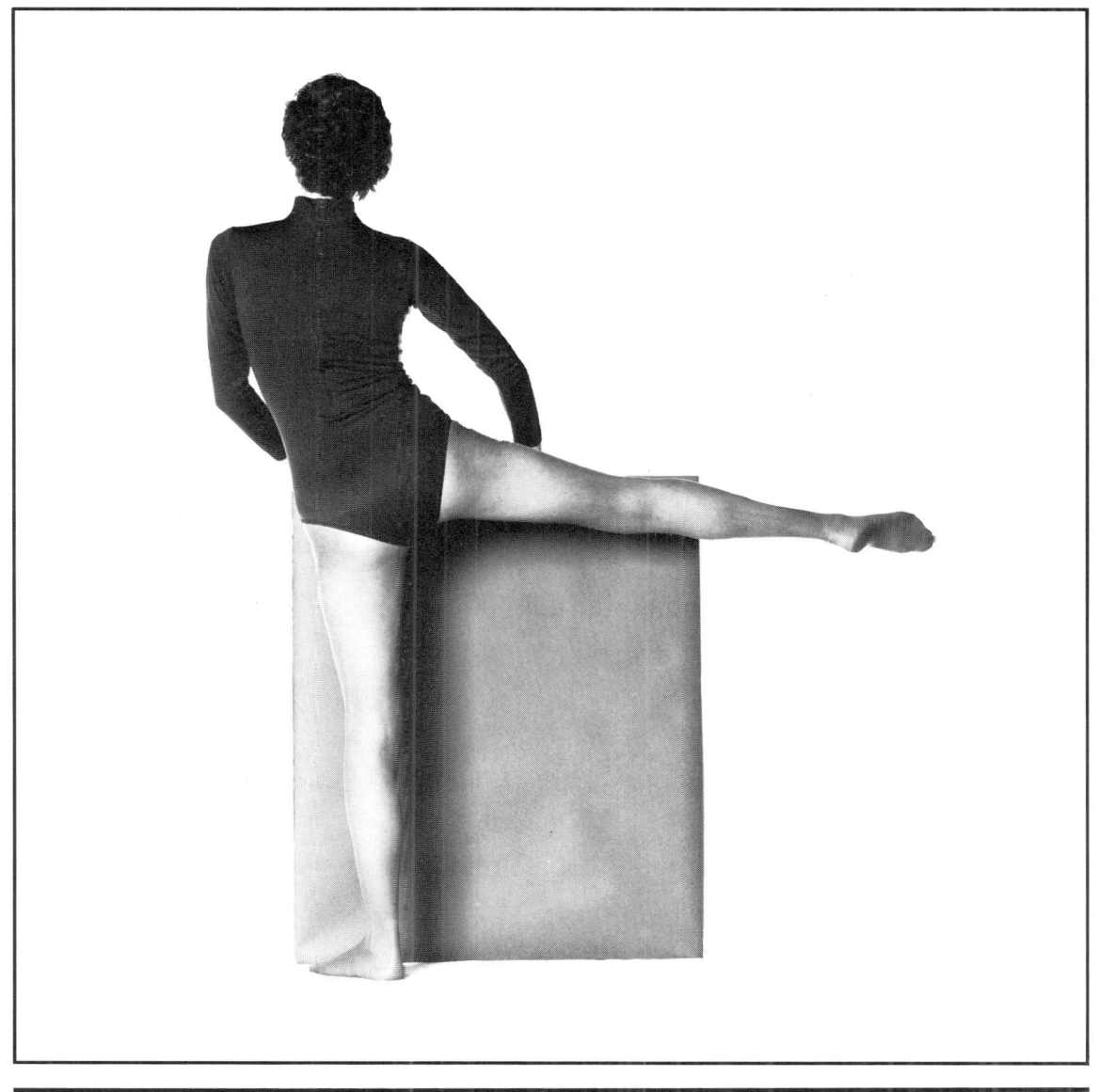

THE BOTTOM IV

This is one of those marvellous exercises which is not only easy to do but works on so many muscles that you really get value for the time you spend on it. It works on your neck muscles, your shoulders, right down your back, and down the backs of your legs. It's especially effective on bottoms. I call it a package-deal exercise!

1.** Lie face down on the floor. Place a cushion under your pelvis. Put your hands down by your thighs and bend your knees so that your feet are pointing to the ceiling.

Lift your head and shoulders off the floor and at the same time lift your knees off the floor.

Stretch your legs upwards and bend again. Repeat this bend and stretch five times. Relax and repeat another five times. Be sure that while you bend and stretch your legs your knees never quite touch the floor. It's by keeping your knees slightly raised off the floor throughout this exercise that will help to give a lift to a sagging bottom.

2. As with all floor exercises involving your back, finish up with the Back Relaxer Exercise, page 46.

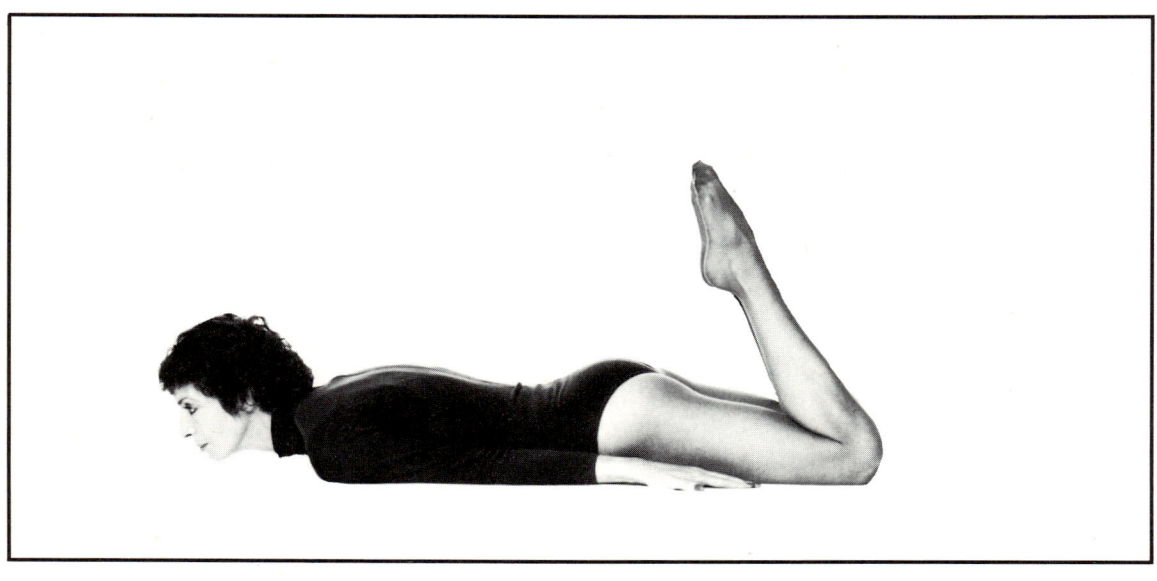

THE BOTTOM 103

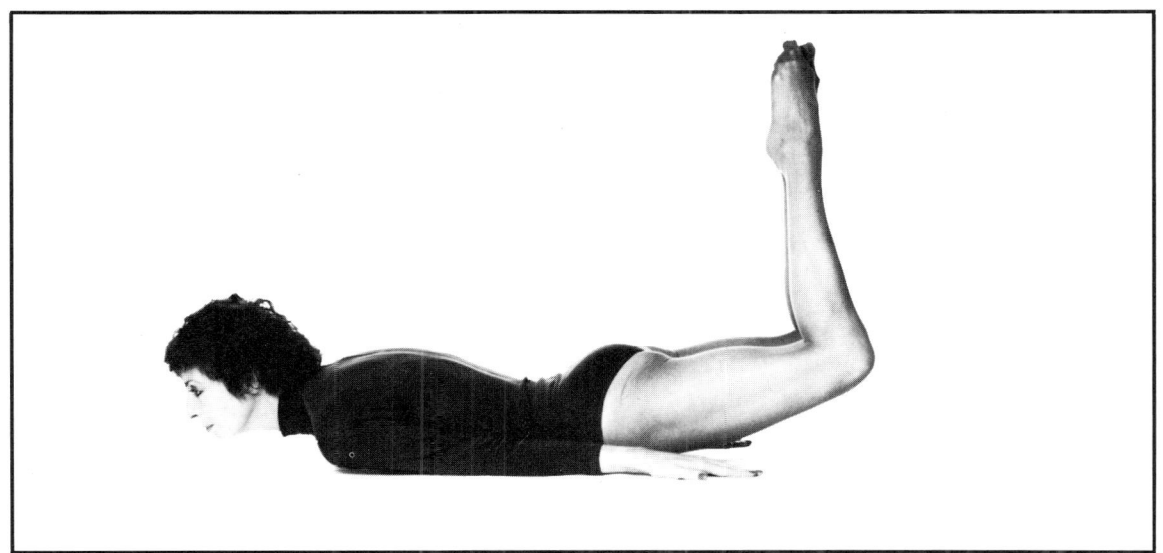

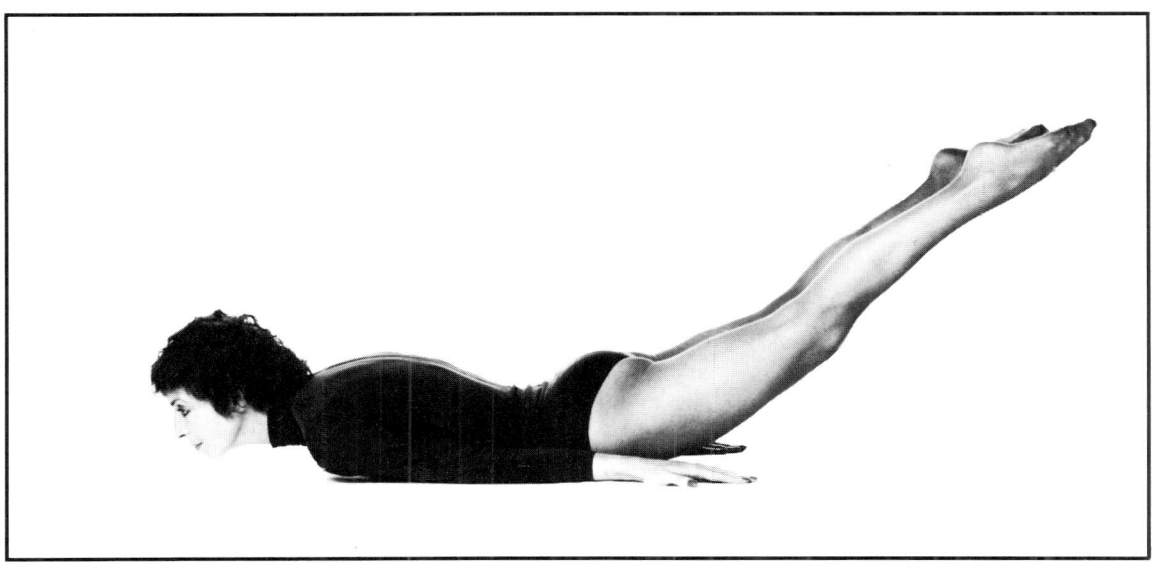

THE BOTTOM V

This exercise is one of the best for stretching and firming all the muscles from your bottom right down the backs of your legs. These muscles need plenty of work as we don't normally stretch them enough during our daily activity. Through lack of use they tend to lose their elasticity which could mean that as we grow older our once natural, and I hope graceful, walk could change to an unattractive shuffle. This exercise can certainly help to prevent this.

1.*** Sit on the floor with your legs together and out-stretched, your toes facing the ceiling. Keep your back straight and upright.

Stretch your arms out in front of you and bend down low. Try to grip your toes with your hands and push your head down to touch your knees. If at first you find this quite impossible try gripping your ankles and pushing your head down. Practise will make this exercise easier. Once you can manage it, stay with your head touching your knees to the count of five. Remember that only by keeping your knees locked straight will you achieve that perfect stretch through the backs of your legs.

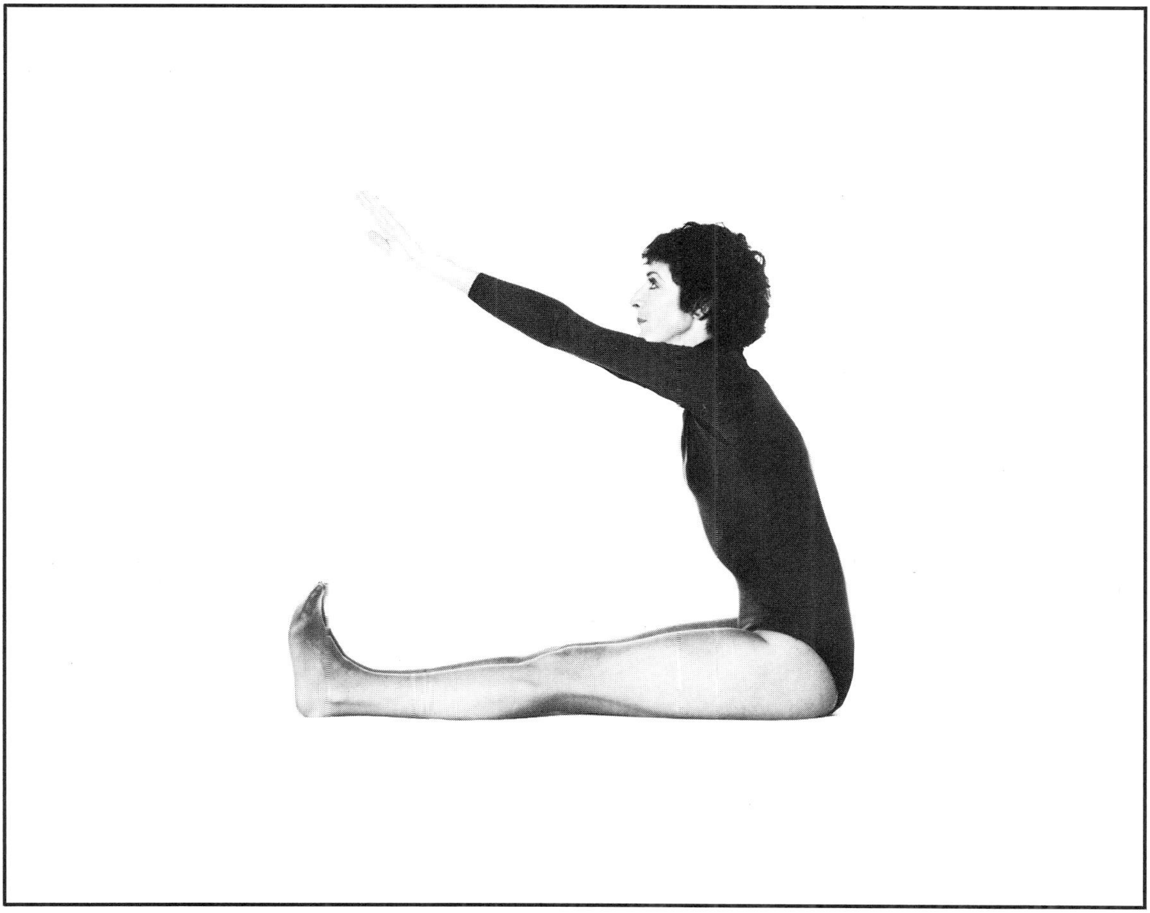

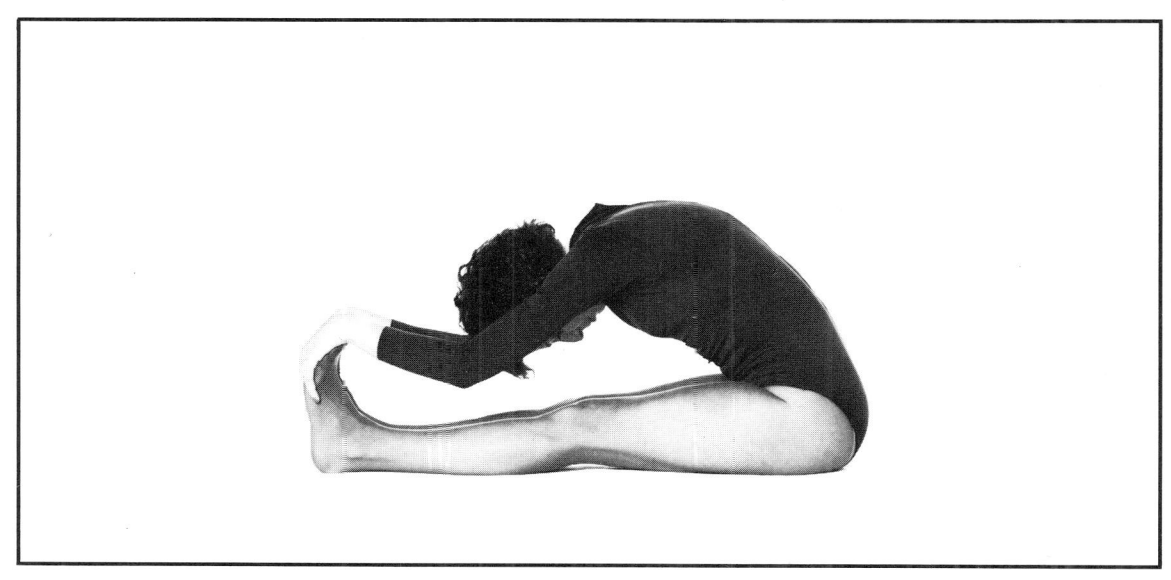

THE LEGS

Legs have some of the longest muscles in your body. Like the muscles in your bottom they are the most coarse, which means that they can be (and should be) exercised vigorously and regularly.

Your leg muscles should be strong to help you carry weights, to help you run fast from danger, to pull, push, jump, and so on. Most people's activities today mean that these muscles aren't worked as much as they should be. And because they're tough muscles, they need tough exercises to benefit them.

THE LEGS I

This exercise strengthens the muscles in the back of your legs, but is also good for your waist and back.

1.* Sit on the floor with your legs spread well apart. Keep your legs stretched. Place your hands behind your head keeping your elbows pushed back.

From the waist lean over to one side. Pump over five times without leaning forward. Come up to a nice sitting position so that your back is straight.

Now lean over to the other side and pump over five times. Keep your elbows well pushed back. And a straight back.

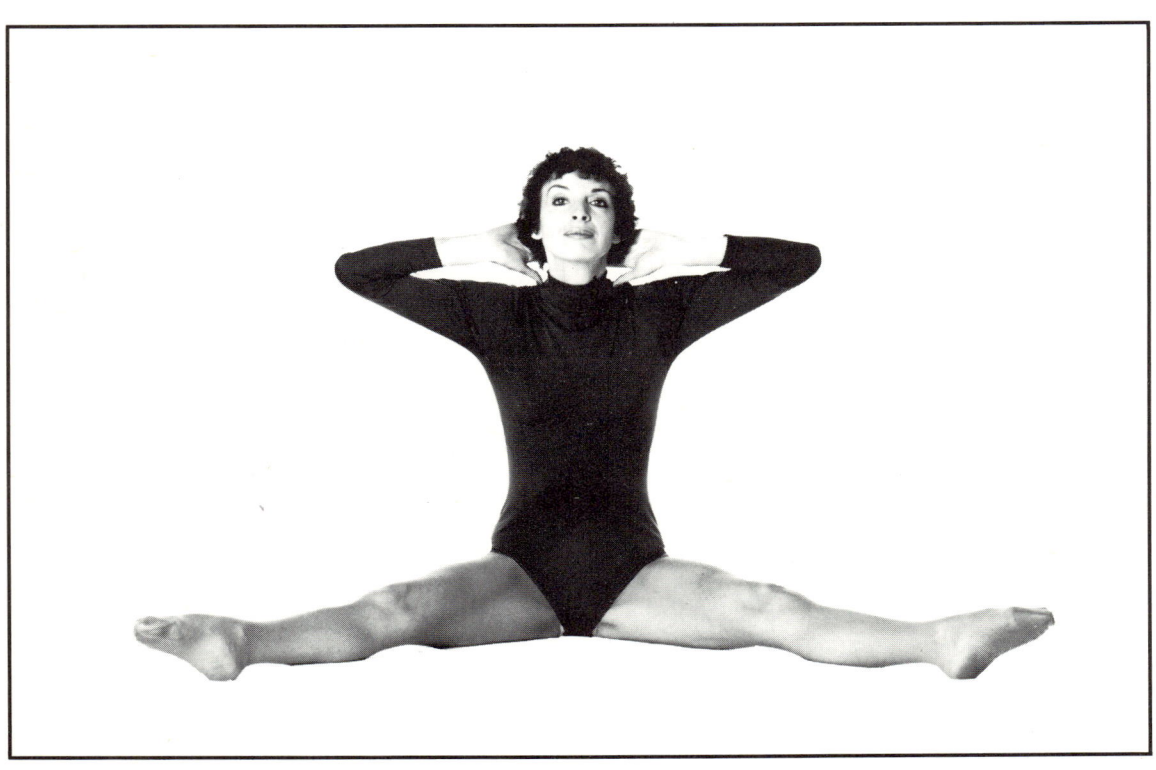

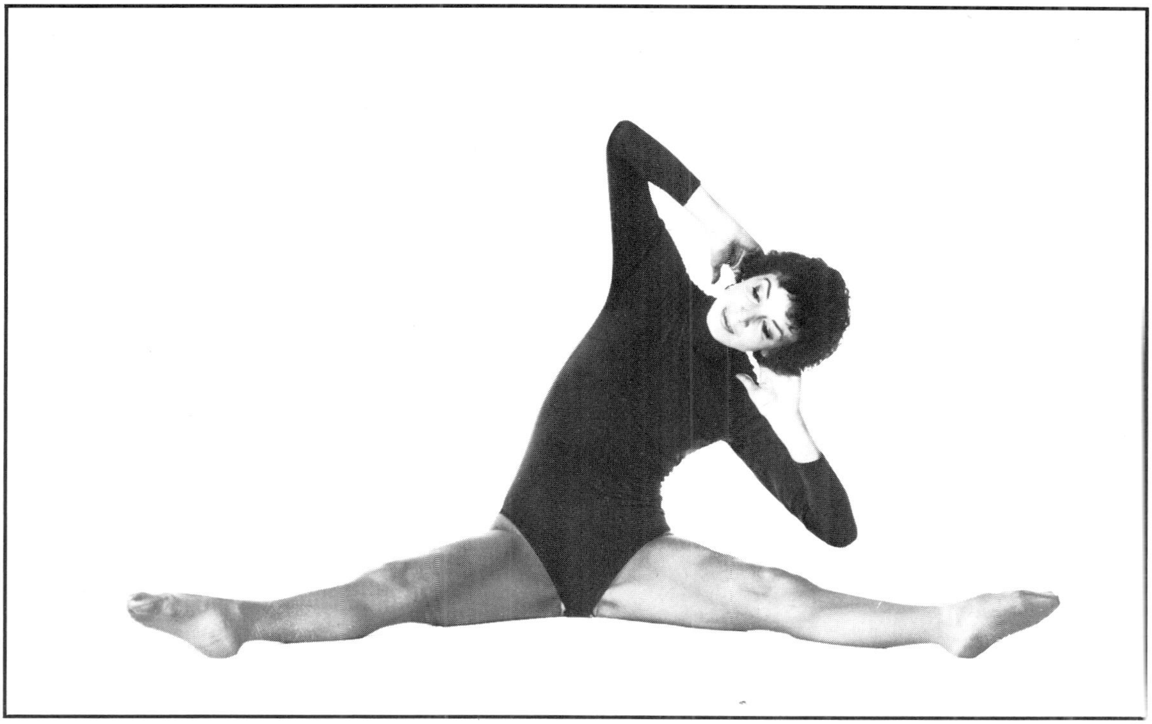

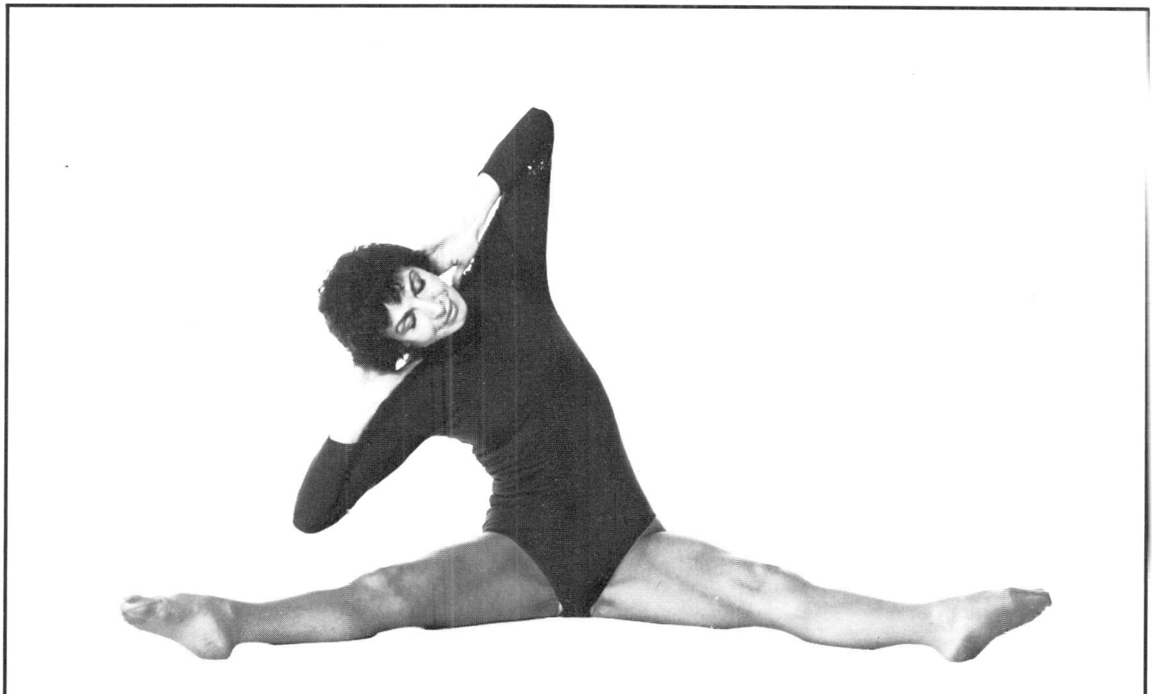

THE LEGS 109

THE LEGS II

This exercise works wonders if you are going on a ski-ing holiday. Start a month before you go and do it daily.

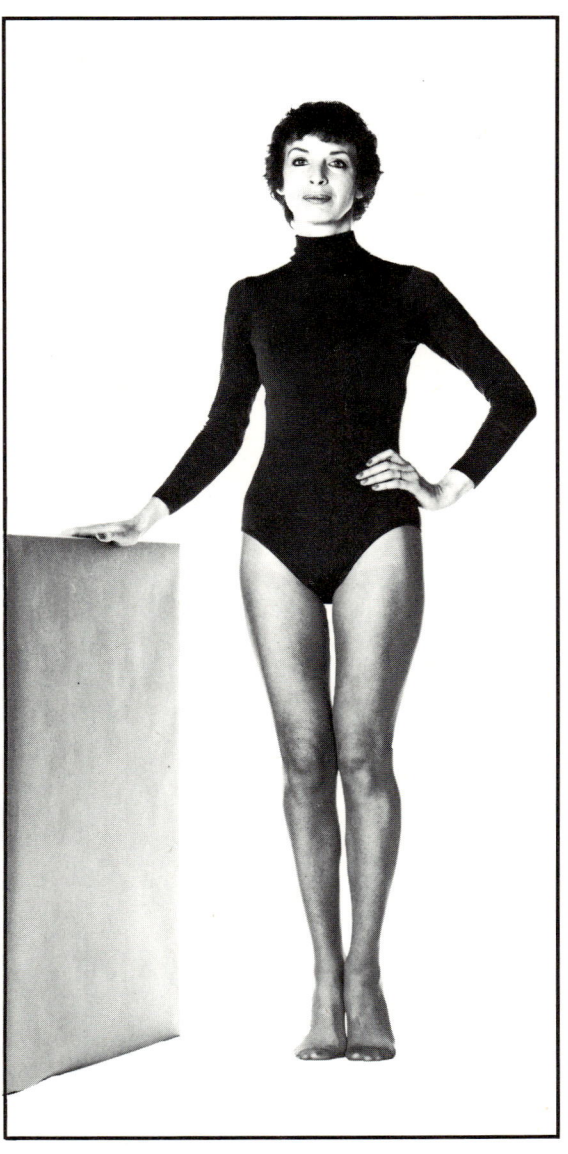

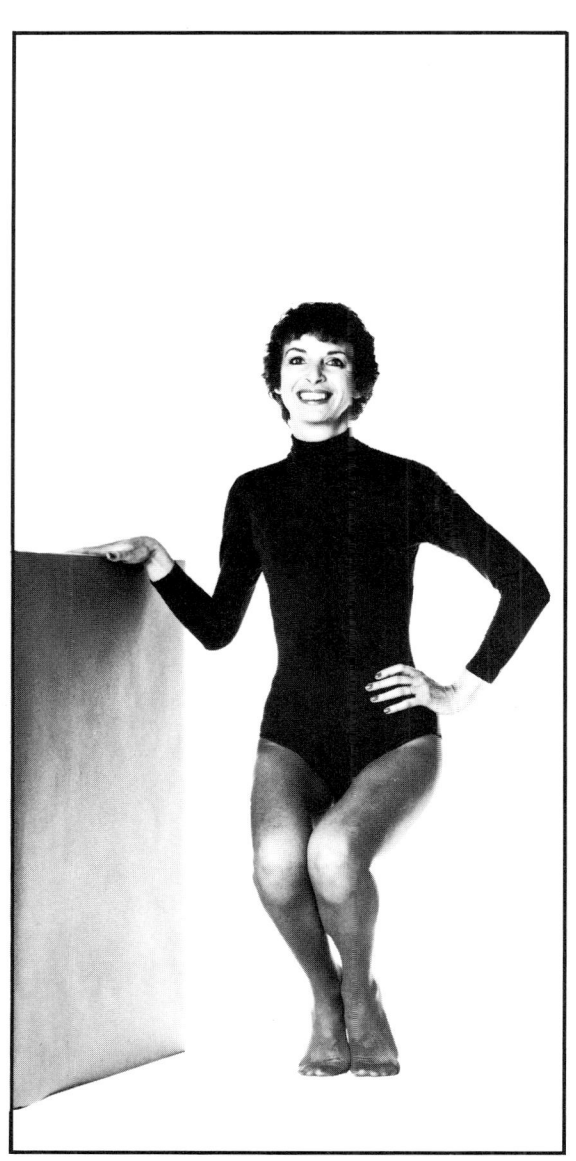

1.** Stand sideways at your kitchen sink for support. Grip the sink firmly with one hand. Stand tall and straight, feet together, and stretch up so that you are standing on the balls of your feet. Stay like this, on tiptoe, for the whole of the exercise.

Bend your knees and lower yourself to the height of a sitting position on a chair. (Your legs can open as you bend your knees.) Hold this position for a count of five and progress gradually to a count of ten. Stretch and repeat.

THE LEGS III

Another package-deal exercise which not merely strengthens and shapes your legs but is also useful as a pre-ski-holiday exercise. It works on your stomach and waist as well.

1.**** Kneel on the floor, knees apart and back straight. You may like to kneel on a cushion although the carpet is usually enough. Lower your head slightly so that you can keep your eyes focused down your body. Place your hands straight down your thighs.

Slowly lean back keeping your spine straight. Your body should be in a straight line from your knees upwards.

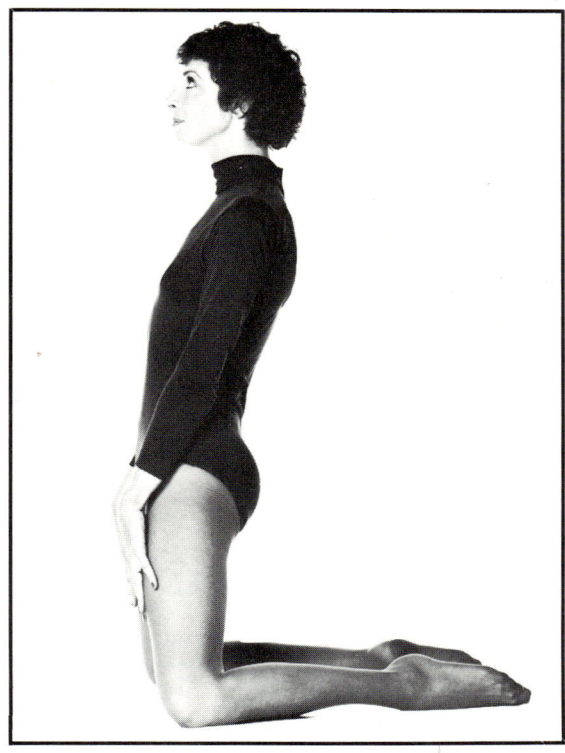

Squeeze your bottom together as though trying to grip a pound note, and move your hips forward as if you have a tail and want to bring it up between your legs. Pull yourself back to kneeling position. Repeat only two or three times at first. You should feel a strong pull in your thigh muscles. Don't let your back take the strain, nor should you pull up from your shoulders. Your thighs take you backwards and your thighs should pull you up.

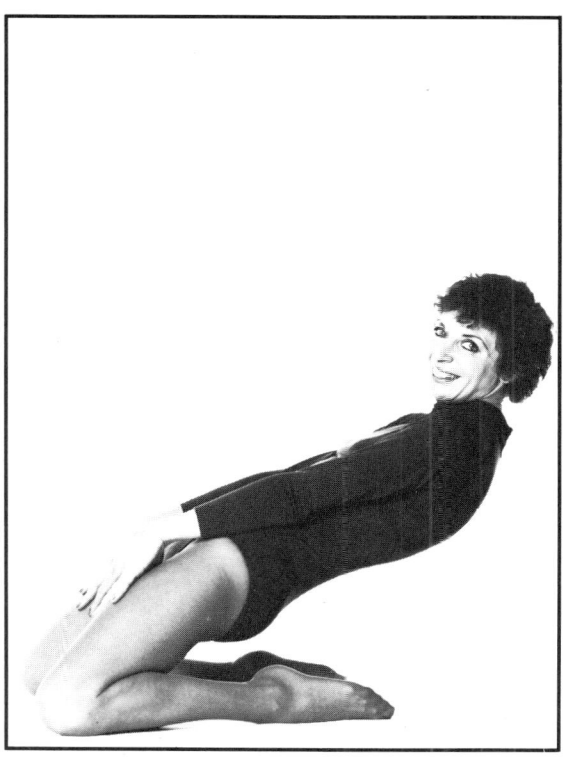
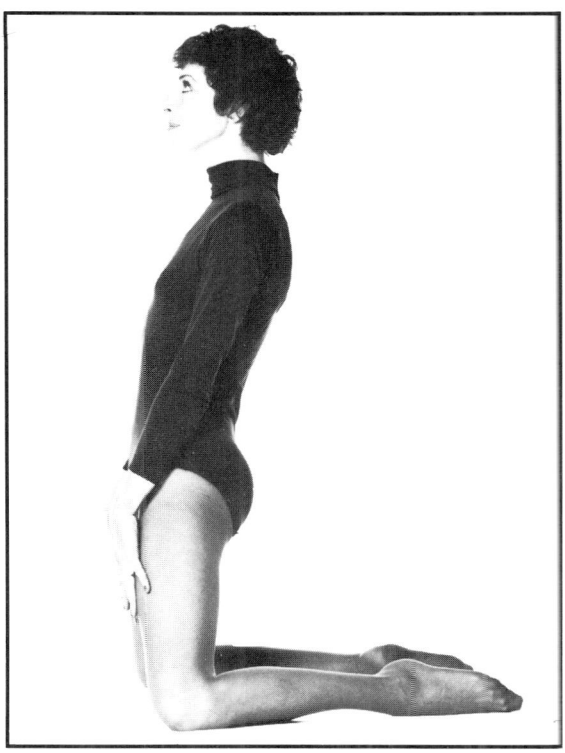

ANKLES AND FEET

Ankles and feet need exercising as much as any other part of the body, and most of us forget about them. If we don't look after them, the joints could cramp up with age and cause us trouble in years to come.

The best rest you can give tired ankles and feet is to lie down and pop a plump cushion under your feet so that they are higher than your head. This gives them the rest they deserve.

Exercise for your feet and ankles will give your legs a lovelier shape and strengthen the muscles for the daily work expected of them while also supporting your weight.

ANKLES AND FEET I

After a day of standing or lifting and carrying, your ankles can become tired and swollen. If you have been sitting for many hours at a stretch, the circulation slows up and your ankle joints stiffen. You need both rest and exercise, which may seem a contradiction, but isn't.

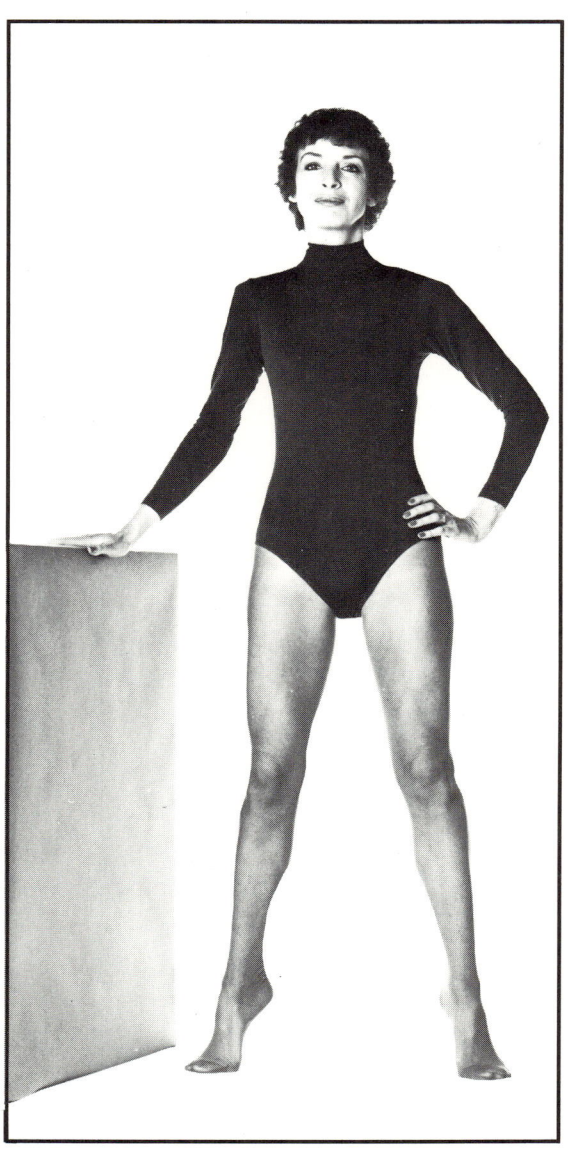

ANKLES AND FEET

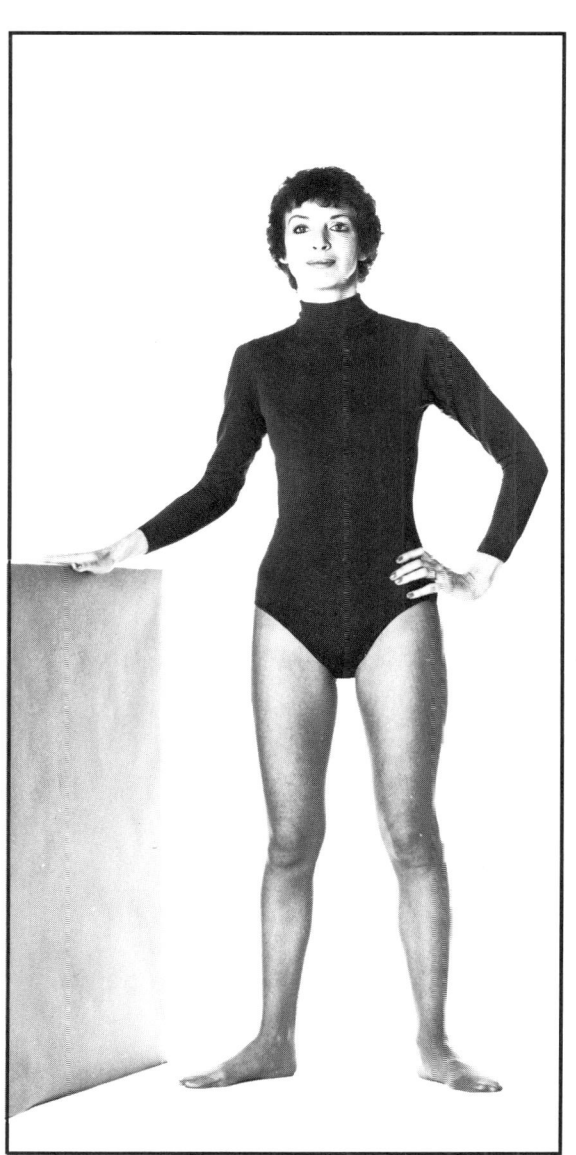

1.* Stand side-ways at the kitchen sink and grip the edge firmly with your hand. Stand with your legs apart. Your body and legs must stay really stiff and straight throughout this exercise.

Rise up onto tiptoes, as high as you can. Now bring your heels down to touch the floor again. You simply keep doing that toe-heel, toe-heel movement faster and faster and try not to stop until you feel a slight ache in your ankles. This will be a good sign, proving that you are really getting your muscles to work.

2.** Even tougher, is to do the previous exercise, but going up and down with one leg at a time. Keep the other leg stretched out in front of you.

ANKLES AND FEET II

We cramp our feet into fashionable shoes which squeeze our toes, or we clonk about on stilts which force the body weight to be borne by parts not meant to. These exercises are good for fallen arches, and tired or flat feet.

1.* Stand tall, barefoot, and put your weight on the outside of your feet with your toes curled round inwards.

Walk round the room like this, on the sides of your feet, at least twenty steps.

2.* Now rise up high on the balls of your feet, bend your knees slightly and walk round the room again.

Alternate the two walks.

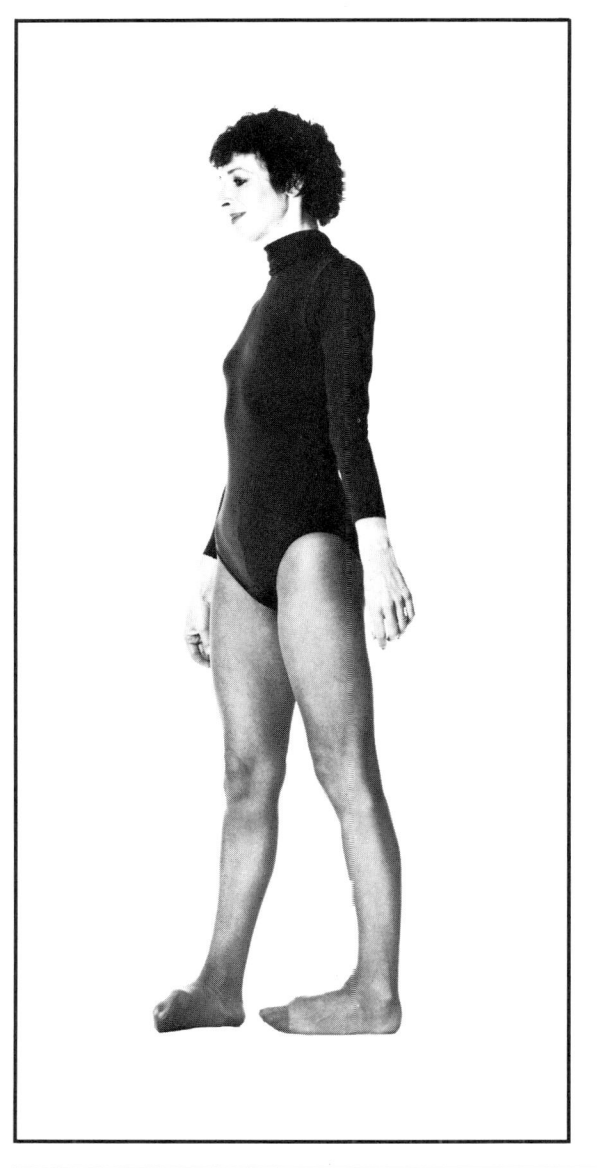 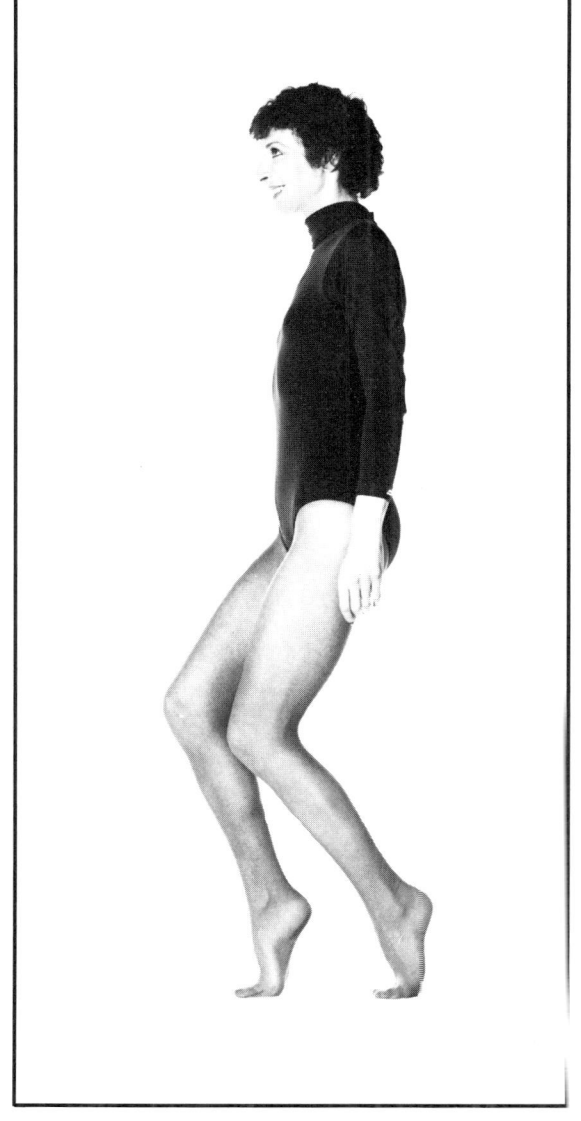

ARTHRITIS

I am glad that research-time and money is being spent on ways to help long-term sufferers of this painful condition, and every year that goes by is a year nearer relief for this problem.

Recent research in Finland suggests that exercise could play an important role in helping to avoid arthritis. It is thought that the cartilage that lines the hip-joints has to be nourished by a fluid which is released when the joint is moved. The more you use the joint, the more fluid is released. So it is not merely sensible to exercise but it is a positive benefit, as it is for our heart and lungs. It can't be stressed enough how much we depend on our physical well-being, and how much that depends on exercise.

ARTHRITIS I

onto your palm as near your wrist as possible.

Open your hand again and curl your fingers back into a tight fist.

Keep repeating these movements and always remember to give your fingers a good stretch before making a fist. Do try to push your fingers down at the end of your palms.

Not long ago I was talking to an eminent physiotherapist who was kind enough to pass on this helpful information for those who suffer from arthritis in the hands. You will need a pair of loose fitting rubber gloves for quick and easy removal, a wash basin or washing-up bowl. Pour in some hot water. Put on your rubber gloves and place your hands in the hot water. Try to keep them in the water until your hands feel good and warm so that the joints and fingers are thoroughly warmed. When you've done this take your hands out of the hot water, remove your gloves and do these exercises while your joints are still warm.

1. Clench your fist as tightly as you can, curling your fingers into your palms. Stretch your fingers out straight. This time stretch your fingers over your palm and press your outstretched fingers down

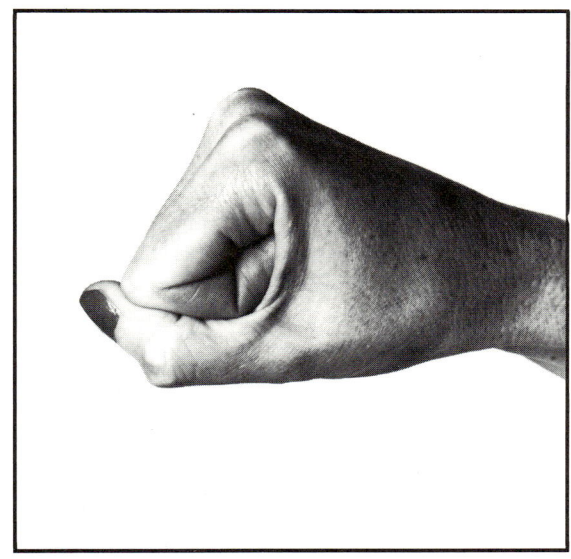

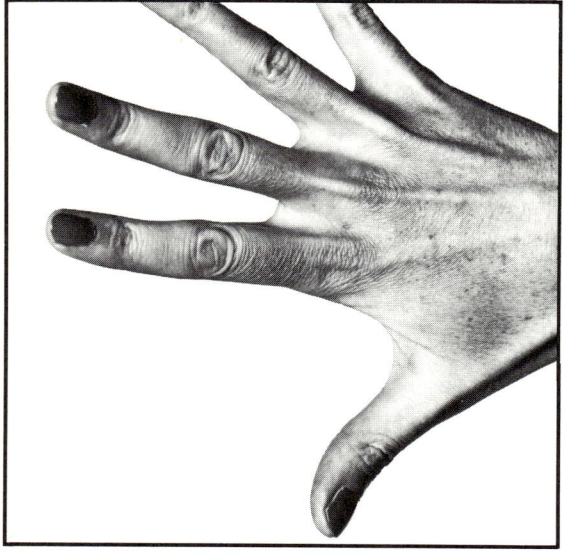

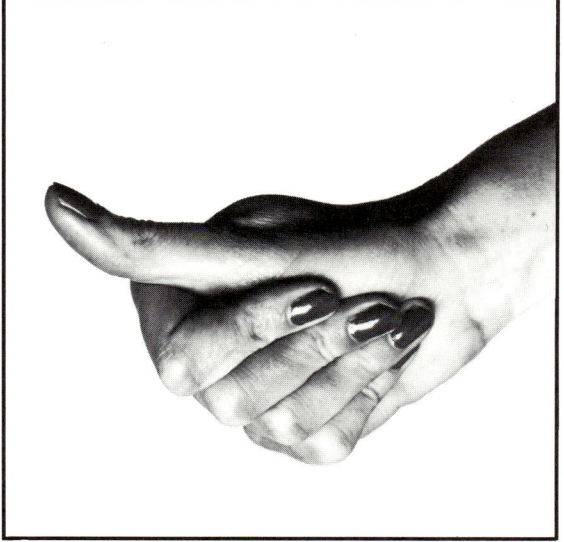

ARTHRITIS II

Should you suffer from arthritis in your hands it usually involves your wrists, so you should try to keep them mobile by doing lots of wrist-circling, as well as the other exercises.

1. Clench your fists tightly keeping your thumb absolutely straight.

Make circles just with your thumbs, keeping them as straight as possible.

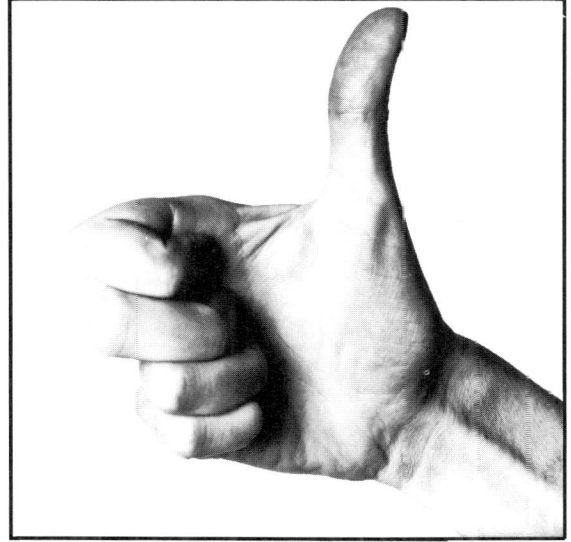

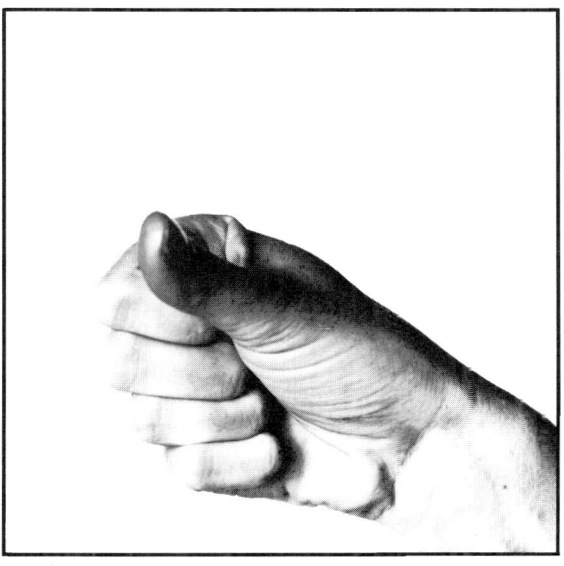

POSTURE

By exercising your body and learning how to use your muscles you will already have become aware of your body, and to some extent your posture should improve. Not only has posture a great bearing on our appearance but it also influences how we feel. Over the years, bad posture can lead to a lot of little aches and pains as well as making one's figure seem worse than it need. By slouching over, whether walking or sitting, you are encouraging and allowing your body to become slack, your shoulders rounded, and your breasts to droop. In some instances poor posture can even push your insides down and this will give you a little pot belly. Inevitably this doesn't do your insides much good, and can lead to backache because you put your natural weight distribution out of balance. Bad posture can also add pressure to your spine and hip joints. And if while walking, you allow your shoulders and head to loll forward you can get headaches, neckaches, and tension around your shoulders.

POSTURE I

It is, of course, difficult always to be conscious of the way you should stand, walk or sit, but having done these exercises regularly I hope you will have become more aware of your body and quite naturally resolve to hold yourself better. (Other exercises throughout the book have, of course, touched upon posture—see pages 33 to 43.)

1. Stand up straight, feet together, and feel really tall. Don't stick your bottom out but rather very slightly tuck in your tail so that your hips have a small forward tilt. Don't thrust your shoulders back, just let your arms and shoulders relax.

Lift your arms out to the sides at shoulder height. Bend your elbows until your hands touch your chest just beneath your chin. Do not allow your elbows to come forward the slightest bit

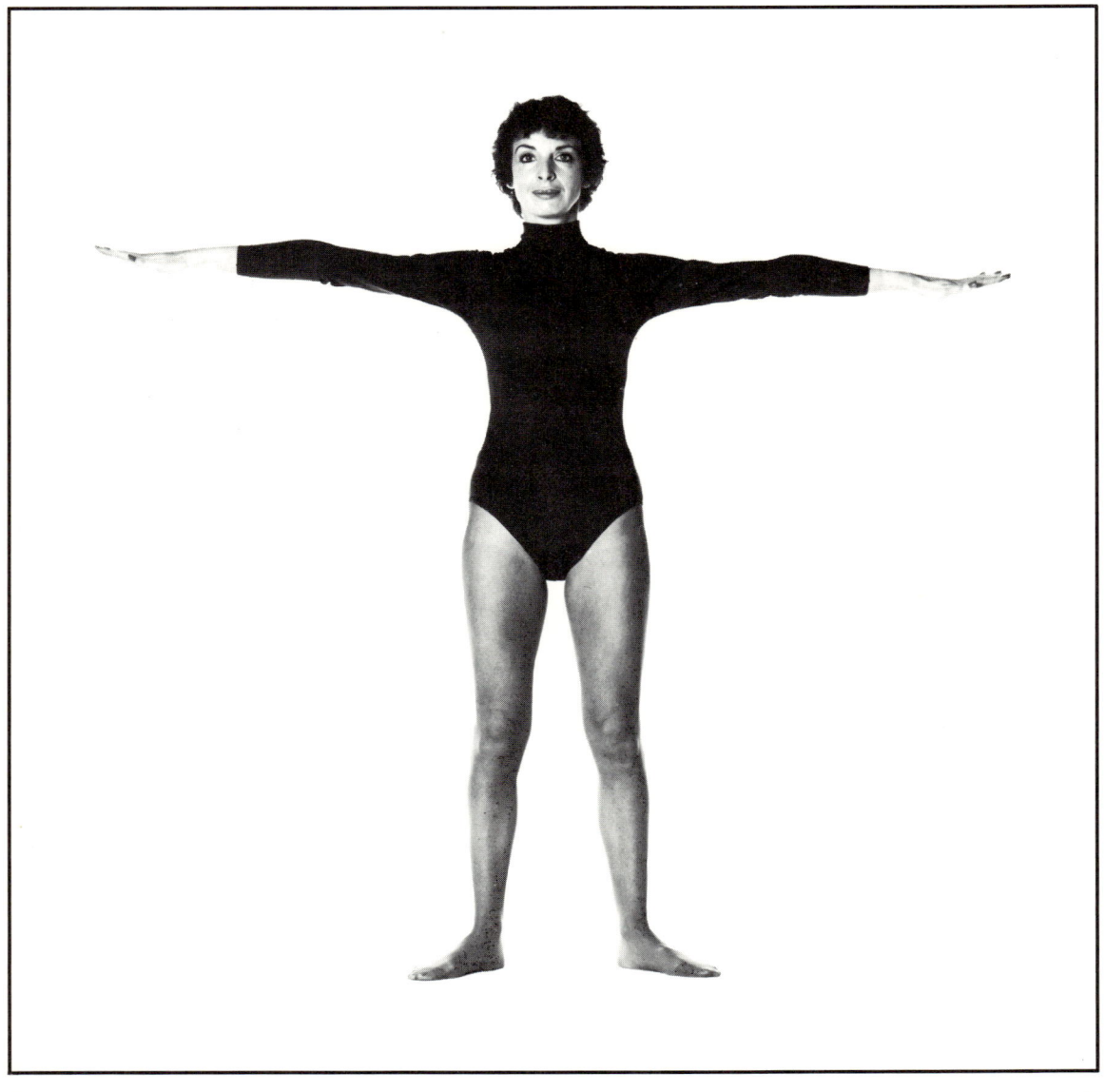

or you will round your shoulders which we don't want. Keep your elbows well out from your shoulders.

Slowly stretch your arms out at either side and then bring them slowly down to your sides. Your shoulders should now be in a correct line to your body. Imagine that there is a bit of string knotted from your head to the ceiling—this should bring your head up a bit without letting it jut forward—and focus your eyes on an imaginary and distant horizon.

Walk forward, tail tucked in, swinging each arm slightly back and forward with its opposite leg. Avoid an army march, with shoulders thrust back too far, bosoms too far out, and bottoms also stuck out too far. What we want to achieve is a nice gliding movement, erect and graceful. See if you can master it. When you are sitting always try to push your bottom into the back of your chair to give you as much support as possible. This is more elegant and comfortable.

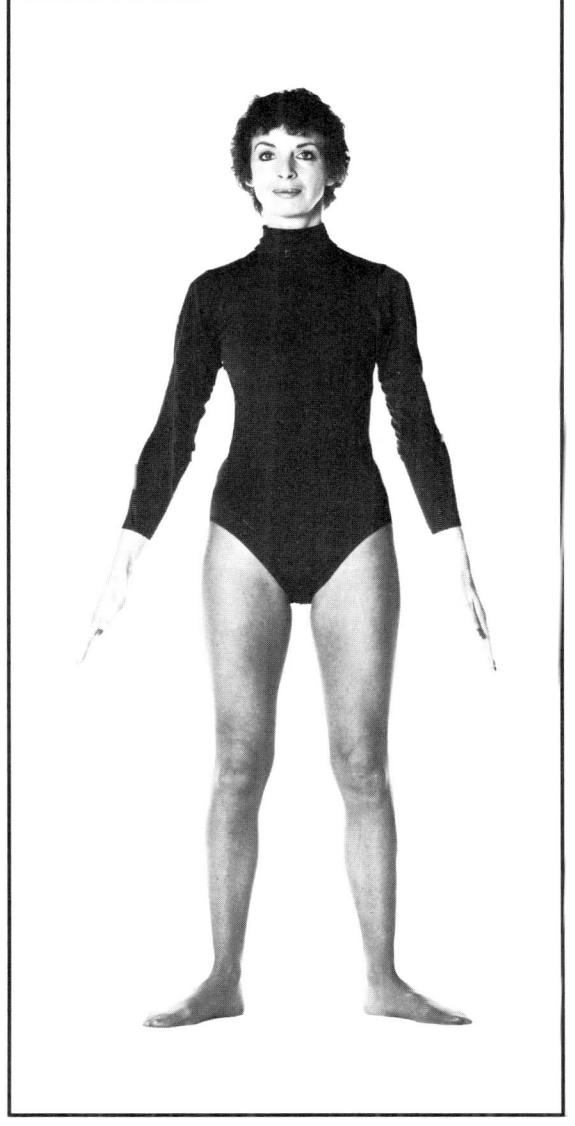

Esther Fairfax runs her own classes in exercise near her home, and also gives exercise sessions at Inglewood Health Hydro in Berkshire. She has broadcast on both local radio and *Woman's Hour*, and has appeared on BBC Television. Esther Fairfax is married to the poet John Fairfax. They have two grown-up sons, and they live in a thatched cottage near Newbury in Berkshire. Esther is in her early forties and, as the photographs on the jacket and inside the book demonstrate, is a perfect advertisement for her philosophy of life.